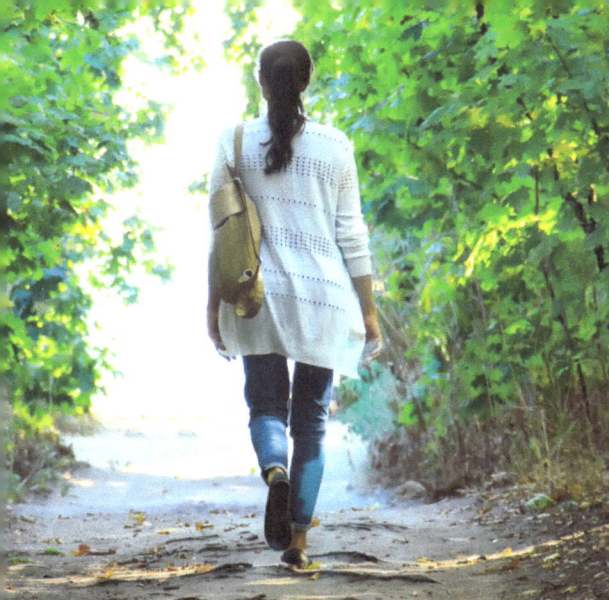

The Migraine Protocol

Free Yourself From Headache Pain

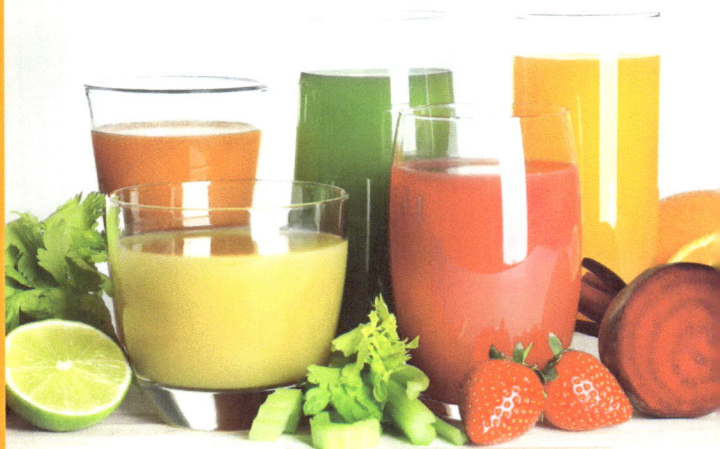

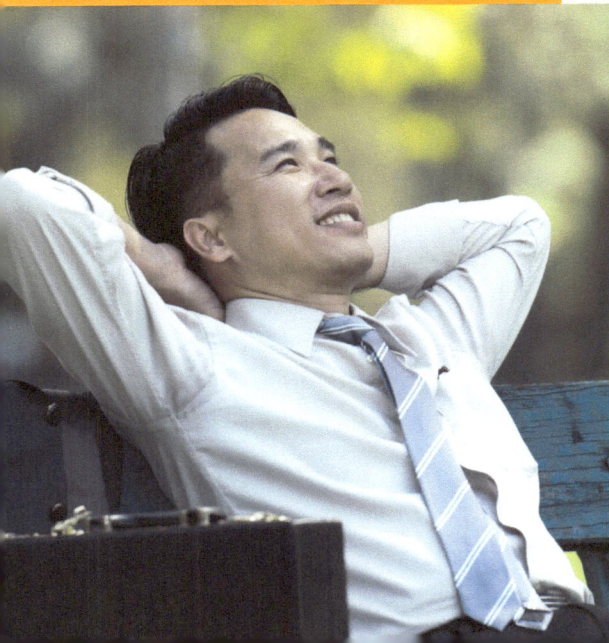

DIANA ANDERSON

The Migraine Protocol
Free Yourself From Headache Pain
Diana Anderson © 2019

Print ISBN: 978-1-61206-193-1
PDF eBook ISBN: 978-1-61206-194-8
Audiobook ISBN: 978-1-61206-195-5

Interior and Cover Design by: Fusion Creative Works, FusionCW.com
Lead Editor: Jennifer Regner

For more information, visit RealMigraineSolutions.com

To purchase this book at discounted prices, go to AlohaPublishing.com

Published by

ALOHA
PUBLISHING

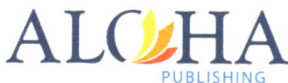

Printed in the United States of America

Disclaimer

The information in this book is not meant to replace the relationship you have with your doctor. This information is a compilation of research along with my extensive personal experience of healing myself from 30 years of head pain. The content of this book is a summary of the alternative and Eastern medicine that resulted in my full recovery, along with some of my story. It is in no way meant to diagnose or give a medical opinion. It is not meant as a professional or medical treatment. I am not a medical doctor.

Keep this in mind and decide for yourself if the information herein is pertinent to you regarding migraine pain.

This is my functional definition of a migraine: a debilitating amount of pain in the head that stops a person from normal living and impacts the ability to do daily tasks. The pain may continually increase until days of bed rest can alleviate it, or a strong medication has covered it up temporarily. This pain interferes with a person's ability to function properly, enjoy life, and may come with other symptoms such as vomiting, nausea, lightheadedness, ringing in the ears, noise and light sensitivity, aura in the eyes, and many other uncomfortable symptoms.

Various doctors and states define migraines differently. For the purpose of this material, it is any head pain intense enough that it interferes with normal functioning.

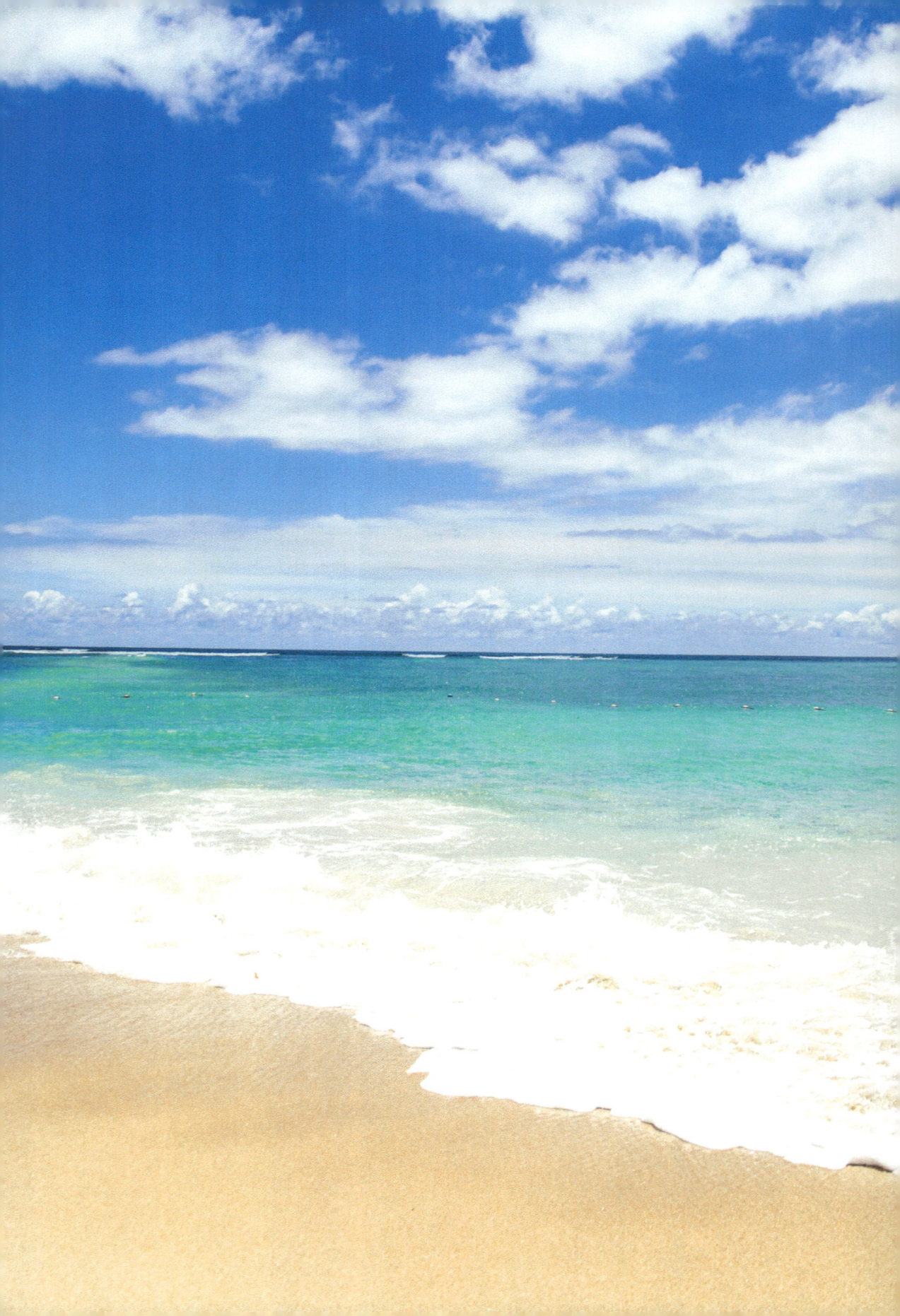

To my family and friends who lovingly supported me through my challenging healing journey, and to the doctors and health professionals who helped me on this path.

If you experience migraines more than eight times per year and they are becoming more frequent, you may have an underlying health issue that is the main cause of your migraines.

CONTENTS

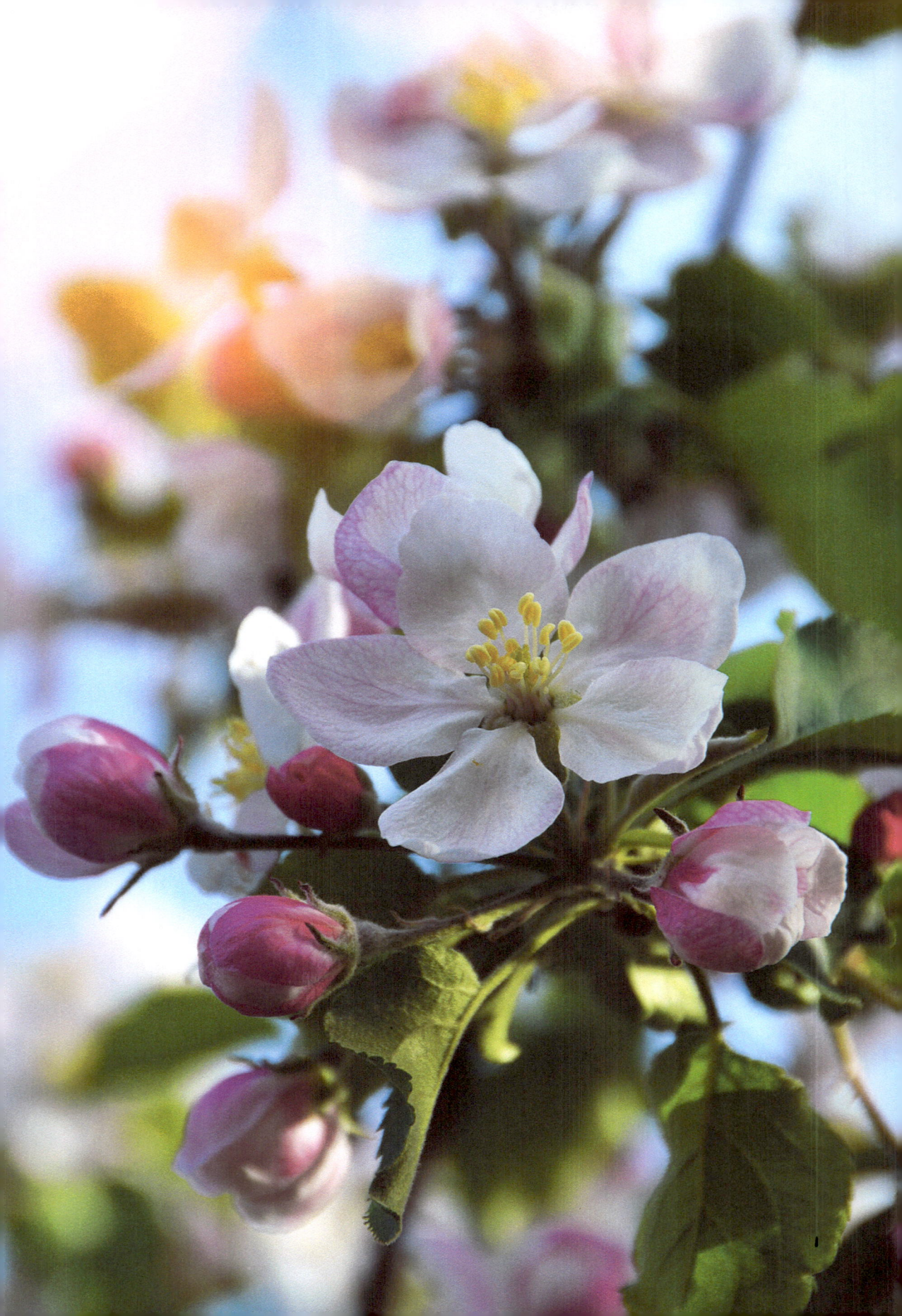

Introduction

All healing of the body involves the physical, emotional, and spiritual. There is no separation.

—Diana Anderson

After suffering from migraines for my entire adult life—over 30 years—I healed myself of headache pain. The most critical thing I learned on my healing journey is that a migraine is a call for help from the body. Giving it what it needs will make that headache go away. Taking a painkiller does not provide what the body needs—and in fact those drugs can make the headaches more frequent, and your health in general worse.

Twelve percent of the worldwide population suffers from migraine headaches. In 2020, this is projected to be a billion people. American employers lose more than $13 billion each year as a result of 113 million lost workdays due to migraines. It is the third most debilitating illness in the world,[1] yet migraine sufferers feel alone and helpless.

The standard treatments for migraines in the United States include powerful painkillers and other pharmaceutical drugs designed to provide temporary relief by masking the symptoms. These drugs do not address the physical issues that produce migraine headaches.

Eventually, these drugs may cease to provide relief. This happened to me. At the time, I was experiencing migraines about 25 days out of every month. I had prescriptions for triptans and opiate painkillers, and they were causing me to have more migraines.

I was desperate for relief from my headaches, which were debilitating enough to affect my ability to eat, sleep, see, stand up, drive a car, work, change altitudes, and keep my eyes open. I had three options: suffer severely, die, or heal my body. I chose the latter. I turned to alternative treatments and alternative practitioners and researched the underlying causes of migraines. What worked for me has also worked for many others, and I believe my protocols will work for you as part of your own healing journey.

Migraine symptoms are often due to a *low flow condition* of the blood or nervous system—that is, a reduced flow of the resources your brain needs to function. These resources are oxygen, glucose, minerals, and proper hydration. Your brain also needs the flow of cerebrospinal fluid (CSF) in sufficient amounts.

The reduced flow of resources can be the result of an issue in your organs, blood vessels, the blood itself, the spine, or the neck. Reduced blood flow or restriction of spinal fluid to the brain can result from physical pinching or obstruction, poor liver function, dehydration, or damage to the blood vessels, among others. Hormonal fluctuations and stress can also create low flow conditions. I have identified five basic types of low flow conditions, and before I healed myself, I had them all.

My research and personal experience helped me gain a new understanding of migraines and how to prevent them.

The first step for me was realizing my prescription medications made my migraines worse and more frequent, so I had eliminate them. Next, I had to find other ways to deal with the agony of migraines as I healed myself. The process took time and the headaches became less frequent, but they did not stop until I uncovered the final answer in my healing journey.

I learned that all migraines begin when the body is in a stress response mode—also known as "fight-or-flight" mode.

All migraines happen when you are in fight-or-flight mode.

Your body can be in fight-or-flight mode without your awareness—it isn't only for acute situations when you are frightened or avoiding injury. I had to learn how to get my body to relax and stop that stress response, which directs critical resources away from the brain in an effort to avoid physical injury and protect the body.

Additionally, when the brain is low on CSF, cortisol—a stress hormone—is released to signal distress. Low CSF can put the nervous system into fight-or-flight mode. Learning to release my body from that stress response wasn't easy, and the basic method in Section Two of this book explains how to do it—called "Stop, Drop, Roll, and Smile." For more detail on this valuable method, visit my website at RealMigraineSolutions.com and read my guide, titled *Stop, Drop, Roll, and Smile for Migraine Relief: How to Stop Headache and Migraine Pain Without Drugs.*

The most important thing I learned was that a migraine headache is an emergency message from your brain, signaling that you are lacking critical resources your brain needs.

A migraine headache is an emergency message from your body that you need critical resources.

You don't need a prescription to cover up the symptoms; you must simply give your body what it needs. The first step toward doing that, regardless of which of the low flow conditions you may have, is to shift your body from fight-or-flight mode into "rest-and-digest" mode. The *Stop, Drop, Roll, and Smile* method helps with this.

As I healed and began to feel normal again, my prevalent thought became my passion to help the billion other people on the planet with migraines. I wrote this book because my heart is full of compassion for anyone who has experienced this maddening disease. You don't have to suffer! And you will be healthier as a result.

The first step in your healing process is to determine the source(s) of your migraines—liver issues, head or neck issues, stress, mineral deficiency, or blood vessel damage.

Find out what produces your migraines with the simple Migraine Test that follows. Armed with that knowledge, learn how to heal yourself using the chapters and protocols that apply to you. Imagine your life without headache pain! This book can help you achieve it.

The first step is to determine what your underlying causes are—liver issues, head or neck issues, stress, mineral deficiency, or blood vessel damage.

THE MIGRAINE TEST

Simple Statements to Help You Understand the Cause(s) of Your Migraines

The Migraine Test statements are designed to help you identify the issues contributing to your headache pain. You may be surprised by the patterns that emerge and the aspects of your daily life that are contributing to your headaches. How often your headaches occur is an important clue to the causes, so several of the statements address frequency.

If you experience migraines more than eight times per year and they are becoming more frequent, or if you feel that you have a low-grade headache much of the time, and/or your migraines last for more than 48 hours—you may have an underlying health issue that is the main cause of your migraines. It is not likely to be due to simple stress or lack of hydration. Especially if they are becoming more frequent, you quite possibly have more than one contributing issue.

Please note that if you have headaches but not migraines, these questions may help you understand the sources of your "regular" headaches but do not necessarily suggest that you are at risk for getting migraines. Each person is unique. My methods work for other headaches as well and have helped many people.

If you do have frequent migraines—more than eight times per year, as a rough guide—it is likely that they are caused by more than one underlying issue.

If you have just occasional migraines, then you are more likely to be impacted by just one or possibly two areas.

Regardless of the causes or the frequency of your migraines, the underlying issues are reversible; you can heal yourself, once you understand what your body needs.

DIRECTIONS FOR THE TEST

If the statements below are true for you, record the numeric score(s) listed for each true statement in the chart that follows the test.

For example, if it is true you have had one head and/or neck injury that resulted in whiplash, then in the "H" column, record 10 points in a box in that column. Do this for each statement to find out which chapter(s) and cause(s) of migraines apply to you. Then sum the total for each column.

If your score in any column is 80 or more, this is likely to be an issue for you and you should read the associated chapter for more information.

THE MIGRAINE TEST

_____ During my lifetime, I have taken ibuprofen (Advil, Motrin) 50 times or more. 20L and 20B

_____ I have had one head and/or neck injury that resulted in whiplash. 10H

_____ My first migraine began on a day of emotional stress, anxiety, or trauma. 20S

_____ I have been hospitalized for dehydration once or more in my life. 30M

_____ I have chronic low back pain or a back injury. 20H

_____ I have taken acetaminophen (Tylenol) more than seven days in a week or more than 30 times in my life. 20L

_____ I have tinnitus, ear tightness, pressure, and/or ear discomfort. 10H

_____ I don't eat three or more servings of fruit and vegetables every day. 20M

_____ I have a lot of worries, such as money concerns, family issues, work, or other stresses. 20S

_____ Cheese, alcohol, MSG, chocolate candy, artificial sweeteners, nitrates, skipped meals, or other foods sometimes trigger my migraines. 30L

_____ I have or do drink soda pop (diet or regular), coffee, black tea, and other diuretics on a frequent basis or I have in the past. 20M

_____ I work at a computer screen or an electronic device for a majority of the day. 30S

_____ I have had a concussion. 10H

_____ I have had more than one concussion. 30H

_____ I currently have a stressful job or life. 30S

_____ My migraines nearly always coincide with neck or shoulder pain. 30H

_____ I have taken either decongestants, antihistamines, or similar over-the-counter or prescription drugs for allergies or sinus congestion more than 50 days in my life. 20B

_____ I am not satisfied with the way my life is right now. 30S and 20B

_____ I have tender areas below my ears when pressing on the area. 20H

_____ I eat a lot of processed, prepared foods or restaurant food. 10M

_____ I yawn frequently during the day, especially when my muscles are tight. 20S

_____ I have more than two servings per day of saturated fats, such as any of the following in any combination: nut butter, coconut oil, potato chips, cheese, red meat, butter, lamb. 10L

_____ I have had shingles as an adult one or more times or I have painful, prickling tingling under the surface of my skin on occasion. 20S

_____ I have been diagnosed with low minerals at some point in my life. 30M

_____ My jaw muscles are tight and/or have pain. 20H and 20S

_____ I have taken hydrocodone, codeine, or other opiate drugs more than 10 times. 20B and 20L

_____ I frequently have shoulder, neck, or back muscle tension and/or pain. 20S

_____ I always feel thirsty, even after drinking water. 10M

_____ I have consumed enough alcohol to be drunk more than 20 times. 20L

_____ I have been diagnosed with a liver issue or I am aware I have liver toxicity. 35L

_____ My first migraine occurred following a head or neck injury. 30H

_____ I have taken blood pressure regulation medication for more than two months. 15B

_____ I have dealt with high levels of pressure/demands in my past. 30S

_____ I have combined a pain relief medication and alcohol on one or more occasions. 20L

_____ I have had more than one head/neck injury that resulted in whiplash. 20H

_____ I have restless leg syndrome or have lots of "ticks" or "shocks" in my muscles or nerves as I fall asleep at night. 30M

_____ There are things I do that I don't want to do. I overcommit and it wears me out. 20S

_____ My menstrual cycle can trigger my migraines, either my period or ovulation. 30B and 30S

_____ I have had a neck injury resulting in long-term neck pain, weakness, and/or misalignment. 15H

_____ I have a difficult time getting deeply relaxed. 20S

_____ I have been exposed to pesticide spray, herbicide spray, mold, heavy metals, or other toxic substances in a heavy dose or over a period of time. 10L

_____ I am aware of ill effects due to my exposure to a toxic substance. 25L

_____ I have daily or weekly neck pain due to muscle tension or stress. 10H

_____ I have had heat stroke. 10M

_____ I have no one I can share my problems with, or I keep my worries and problems to myself. 30S

_____ I grind my teeth or hold my jaw tight and have tooth pain or damage to my teeth. 20H

_____ I do repetitive physical work all day. 30S

_____ Often it is difficult to take a slow, deep breath. 30S

_____ I get leg cramps at least five times per year. 10M

_____ I get rebound headaches after taking painkillers or triptans. 30B

Record your points for each question in the correct column by letter. Put the sum of your points for each column in the bottom row of the chart.

MIGRAINE PROTOCOL

L	H	S	M	B

WHAT'S NEXT?

For any column with a total of 80 or greater, read the chapter in Section 2 that coincides with each of those columns:

L: Chapter 1 – How Poor Liver Health Causes Headaches

H: Chapter 2 – Head and Neck Injuries Can Lead to Headaches

S: Chapter 3 – Stress Affects Your Body's Systems and Your Health

M: Chapter 4 – Minerals, Oxygen, and Hydration Are Critical Resources for Brain Function

B: Chapter 5 –The Circulatory System Must Be Healthy to Prevent Migraines

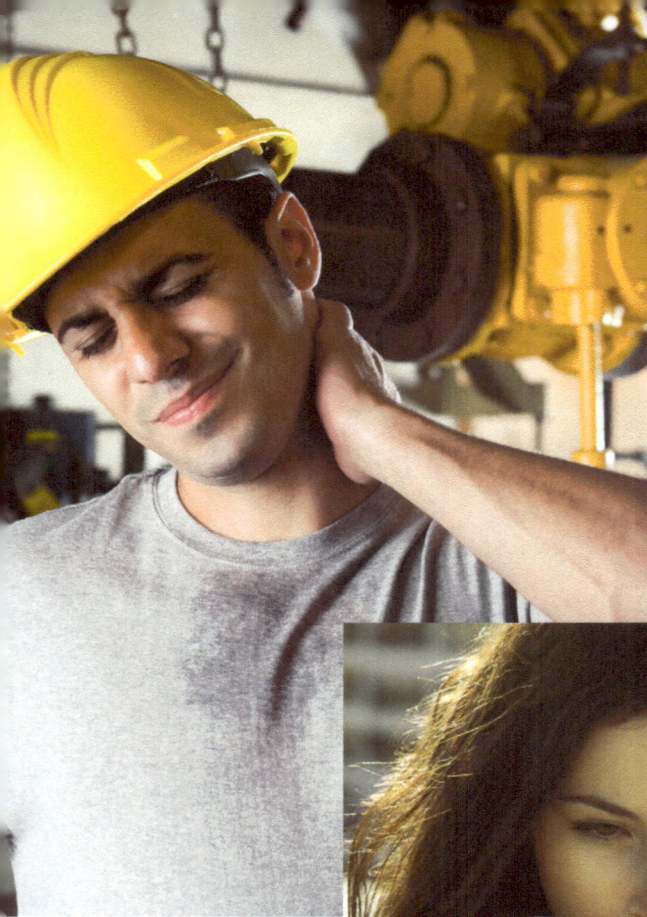

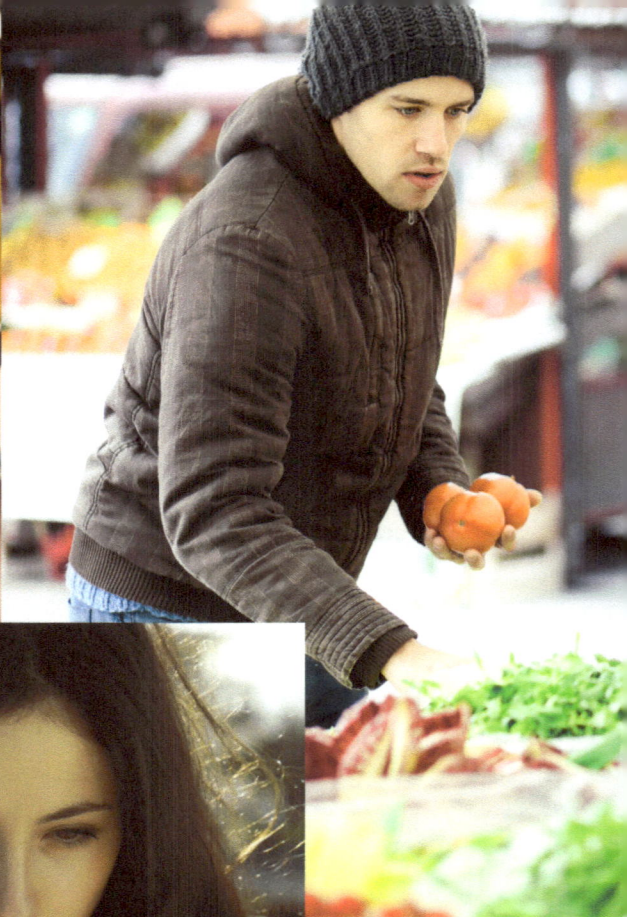

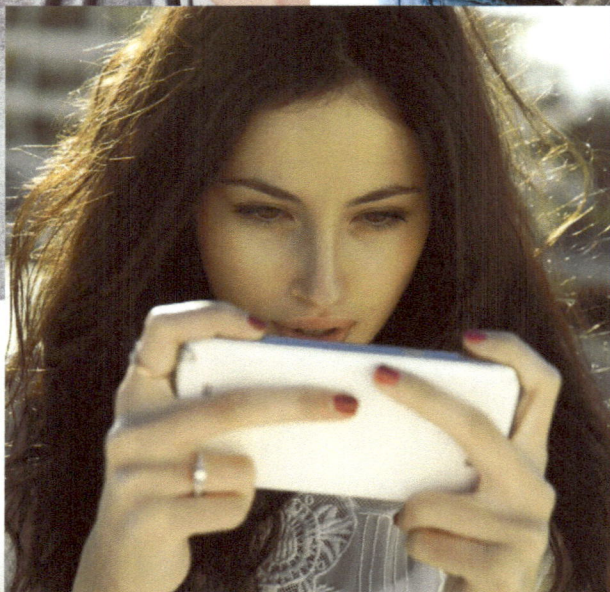

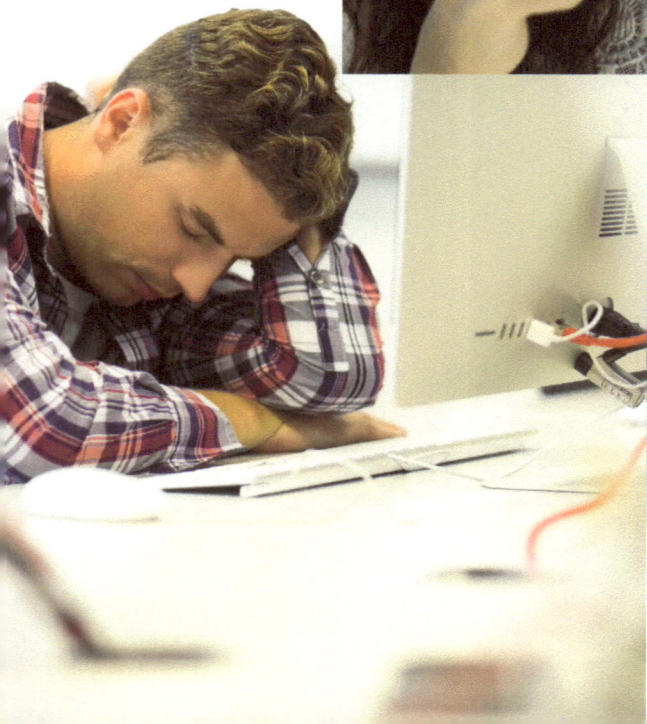

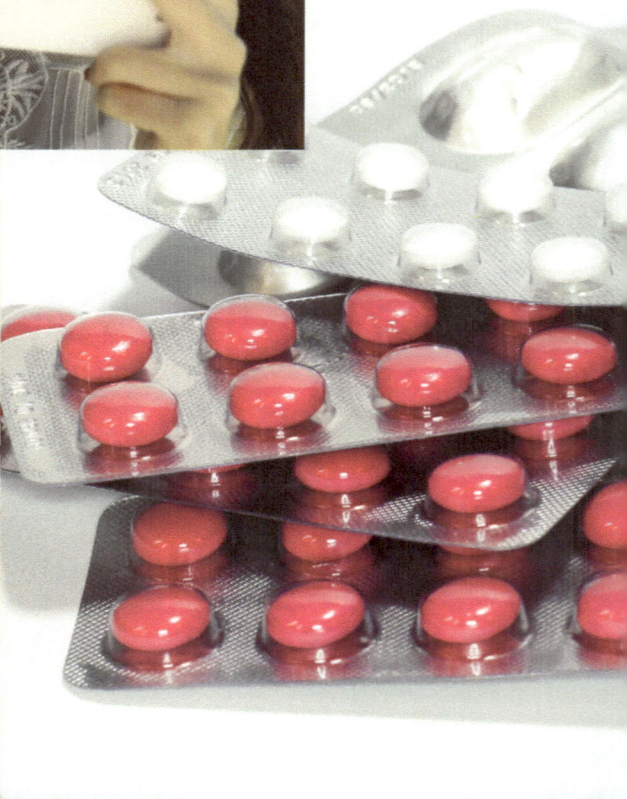

SECTION ONE

Understand the Five Underlying Causes of Low-Flow Migraine Headaches

Although migraines may seem to develop randomly, they are actually caused by specific issues and are not random at all.

Migraines are a signal from the nervous system, screaming for resources that are being redirected to other areas of the body. This happens because your body is locked in a fight-or-flight response or has a low flow condition—wherein resources are limited due to health issues.

Lack of resources to the nervous system means that not enough blood—loaded with oxygen, hydration, glucose, and minerals—is reaching the brain and nervous system. It can also mean that you don't have enough movement of cerebrospinal fluid (CSF)—or enough fluid, period. CSF carries all of the resources that are critical for your brain's function.

Your brain requires CSF at all times. Your body produces CSF all day long, nearly a liter a day, in two ways. Most of it is created by the *choroid plexus,* which is a network of special capillaries in the ventricles of the brain that convert the plasma that is delivered by the blood into CSF. The second way you make it is through cells within the brain secreting the liquid from the cells. If your blood can't deliver adequate nutrients in the plasma, either due to dehydration, thick blood, or inflammation, then the brain hurts from lack of sufficient CSF. When CSF is low from dehydration or something else, headaches result and cortisol is released in the brain as a stress signal, causing the nervous system to go into a state of fight or flight. Frequently this results in reduced tolerance for pain, and nausea.

When the needed resources are not provided after the screaming pain begins, the brain will force a shutdown to preserve the nervous system, leaving you unable to function and forcing you to rest. It is certainly a cry for help, and help can be found when oxygen and blood are abundantly directed and are able to reach the central nervous system.

Part of understanding the causes of your migraines is knowing the frequency and duration of your headaches.

- For a person with occasional migraines, the most likely cause is an extended time in the fight or flight response, also called the stress response. When you are in this state, your body directs resources away from the brain to the muscles in large amounts. This depletes the resources and also diminishes the brain's supply.

- For a person with more frequent migraines, the most common cause is a taxed or stagnant liver, which has been damaged by many possible factors.

Multiple causes are also common for a person who suffers from more frequent migraines. For the sufferer with tremendous neck or back pain with migraines: neck, brain stem, and back injuries, as well as gross misalignments of the spine, can interrupt the flow of blood, spinal fluid, and nerve flow to the head. These issues can be a huge contributor to the lack of resources. Additional stress or blood vessel damage from long-term use of over-the-counter (OTC) or prescription medications can then throw the system out of balance much easier.

1

How Your Liver
Protects Your Brain

Liver toxicity is a contributor, if not *the* cause, for many types of headaches—and especially migraines. Of the 500-plus functions of the liver, several of the major roles are primarily to keep the brain functioning properly and to supply it with resources.

An example of how the liver impacts a headache is a hangover, when a taxed liver is unable to deliver needed resources to the brain and body because of the large amount of alcohol it must process. While the liver is busy detoxifying the body of excessive alcohol, the blood cells are not refreshed by the liver and can't keep up with the demand for the nutrients the body needs—especially hydration.

If you scored 80 or higher in the L, M, or B columns, this chapter applies to you.

LIVER FUNCTIONS

Toxin Removal

The liver cleanses your blood cells and plasma of toxins. Your blood cells are like tiny buses, loading nutrients and delivering them where they are needed. Oxygen from the lungs, and minerals and vitamins from the digestive system are carried in the blood cell buses. Blood also transports toxins from the capillaries as they draw out waste and bring it back to the liver and lungs to be excreted. If the toxins aren't removed from the blood cells, the blood has reduced capacity for delivering nutrients.

An unhealthy or overloaded liver can't clean the blood sufficiently, which causes the blood cells to be inflamed, sluggish, and toxic. They can't carry oxygen as well, in this state. Lack of oxygen and nutrients to the brain are major causes of migraine pain. When the liver is overtaxed, the entire body is affected with lower levels of oxygen, but the brain is most vulnerable. This knowledge is well-known in traditional Chinese medicine but is not regularly recognized in Western medicine.

Nutrient Storage

Your liver stores the vitamins, minerals, and glycogen (the body's storage form for glucose) for fuel to the body, brain, and nervous system. When your body is low on any of these substances, a healthy liver will push these directly to the brain, bypassing other organs of the body.

Your liver also produces certain proteins for blood plasma so it can carry minerals, enzymes, and hormones to the cells, including brain cells.

TOXINS AND THEIR IMPACT ON BLOOD AND LIVER

We are all exposed to environmental toxins we can't see or identify. Sometimes they are detectable by smell, but often you can't sense them. There are external toxins that compromise the liver and circulatory system, reducing blood flow and oxygen delivery.

Your body is equipped to handle and expel toxins. We all deal with unrecognized toxic compounds, natural and manmade, that are harmful to the body on an ongoing basis. It is unavoidable in the modern world. A healthy body is able to process the toxins through the liver and eliminate what is not wanted or useful. However, a body with a compromised liver or circulatory system, or with poor flow of blood and lymph to and from the head, will be more impacted by mold, chemicals, and other toxin exposure than a healthy person whose liver and lymph system are eliminating contaminants well. Chronic exposure to high levels of toxins can also create stress for the body's detoxification pathways.

Mold

One of the most harmful pollutants is mold. Exposure to toxic mold reduces oxygen supply in the body in several ways. Foremost, it taxes the liver, as the liver has to work to rid the body of the harmful substance. The liver and the natural defense system spend energy ridding the body of mold and as a result, the liver doesn't have the available resources to clean the blood fully of all poisons, leaving the blood cells "congested" and less able to carry oxygen and nutrients.

Mold exposure triggers immune responses which cause inflammation, as white blood cells attack the foreign invader. Extra waste, white blood cells, and toxins pollute the bloodstream, interrupting the flow of oxygenated liquid to the cells and tissues and clogging the system. This can lead to other circulatory problems along with arthritis, headaches, and high blood pressure.

Medications

Pharmaceutical drugs play a major role in liver damage and toxicity. You may or may not be able to see this damage with normal blood tests, so you must look to the secondary symptoms I have listed to identify the liver as one of your headache causes. Long-term, consistent use of OTC or prescription medications can overtax the liver. *This includes medications prescribed for migraines.*

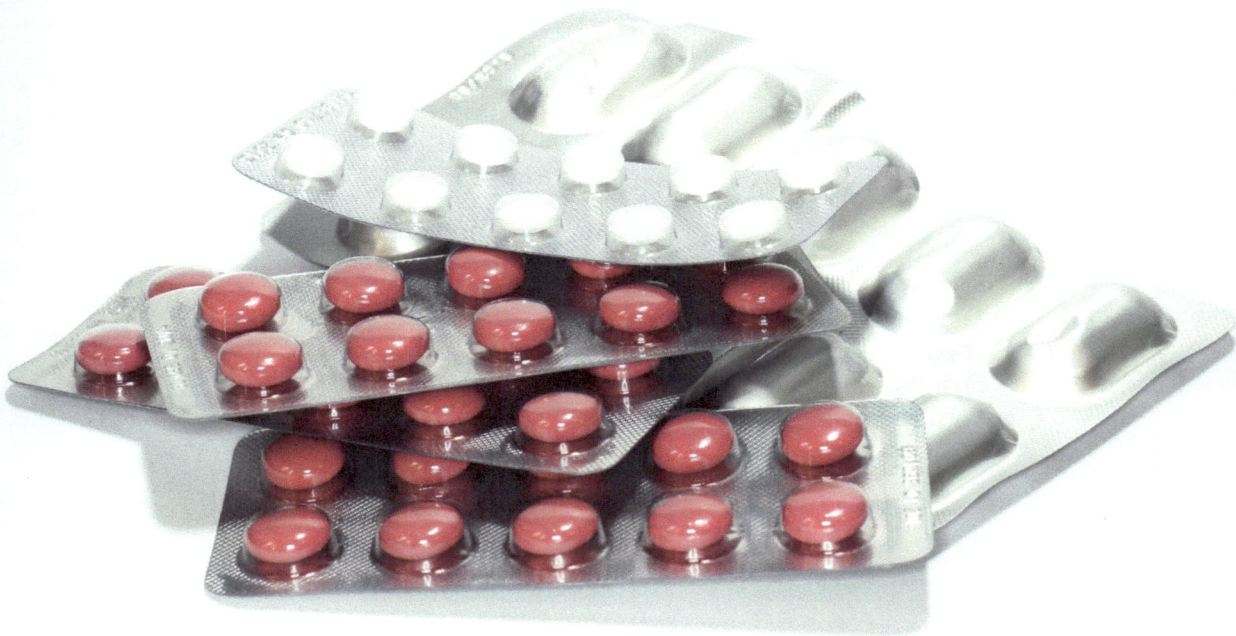

Other Toxins

In addition to mold, other toxins that affect the liver are listed below:

- Radon

- Cigarette smoke

- Wood smoke

- Dust

- Asbestos

- Mercury/heavy metals

- Radiation

- Pesticide sprays

- Chemicals for cleaning

- Herbicides and pesticides

- Processed food

- Soda

- Alcoholic beverages

Parasites

Parasites are another potential hazard to your liver and body functions. If you travel abroad, eat any raw fish or meats, or drink water from mountain streams, you can ingest a parasite, which can greatly impact your liver and digestive function. This is another area where professional help is recommended. This is not a specialty of Western medicine so you can turn to Eastern medicine, traditional Chinese medicine, or other natural practitioners such as naturopaths. Please be careful. There is a lot of bad advice from nontraditional practitioners, some of whom are well meaning but don't have the credentials to treat parasites. Stay with reputable health practitioners who have the experience to help you heal from unwanted bugs.

It is critical to restore the liver to proper function. If the liver is not able to clean the blood from toxins and store glycogen, vitamins, and minerals for the brain, migraines will continue.

Be aware that regardless of your level of health and circulation, when the body flushes out toxins, it also flushes minerals. Anytime you are exposed to contaminants, you need to also replenish the lost minerals. See the chapter on minerals for more details.

Possible Symptoms of Poor Liver Function

Any of these symptoms can indicate an issue with the liver, however, they may be caused by other issues too. Having several of these symptoms can definitely point to a sluggish liver.

- A change in sensitivity to caffeine or medication
- Hyper pigmentation on the skin
- Skin problems (acne, rashes, or psoriasis)
- Difficulty with fatty foods (nausea, headaches, or heartburn)
- Excess body odor
- Food allergies and sensitivities
- Tendency to bruise easily
- Waking up at 2 a.m. or 3 a.m. for no reason
- Pain predominantly on right side of head
- Bitter taste in mouth
- Excessive thirst
- Poor digestion, nausea
- The blood pressure rises with stress
- Constipation
- Poor appetite
- Dry, cracked nails
- Sensitivity to perfumes, scents, smoke, and other smells
- Food triggers for your headaches

Many people will never have a headache triggered by cheese or peanut butter. However, if you have low blood flow for one or more reasons, then peanut butter, bacon, or coconut oil could send you over the edge into a headache due to increased blood viscosity, adding to the problem of reduced blood and oxygen delivery. See the list of blood-thickening foods in the Appendix.

> ## If cheese, alcohol, saturated fats, or MSG trigger your headaches, poor liver function is a factor in the cause of your migraines.

Fats

Your liver produces bile, which carries away waste and breaks down fats in the small intestine during digestion. It you are eating saturated fats such as cheese, chocolate, or lots of butter, an overtaxed liver will struggle to break down these fats. These foods cause blood viscosity to increase, making the blood cells less efficient at delivering supplies, and a headache can result.

THE LYMPH SYSTEM AND THE BLOOD WORK TOGETHER

The circulatory system and lymphatic system rely on one another. When your blood is not circulating well, this affects the lymph system. The lymph system provides critical interstitial fluid to fill the spaces between cells and within tissues, to provide nutrients to the cells while also picking up waste products. Your blood vessels and lymphatic vessels circulate fluid into and out of surrounding tissue so the fluid can be drained.

Tiny lymphatic capillaries present in the tissue draw in interstitial fluid, where the fluid becomes known as *lymph*. Lymph travels through the lymphatic capillaries, which join at lymph nodes, where the lymph fluid is filtered. The lymph system ultimately drains into the blood circulatory system.

When the lymph is working correctly, extra fluid is eliminated from the body, which stops tissue from swelling or puffing up. However, when you are sick, injured, or have tight muscles and poor circulation, fluids build up in the damaged area, which is why throbbing, swelling, and pain occur.

Many solid materials also get picked up by interstitial fluid, including pieces of dead cells, pathogens such as bacteria and viruses, and even tumor cells. When the lymph system can't circulate due to tight muscles and poor blood flow, the system gets backed up. This fluid backup causes pain, which worsens a headache. It also causes inflammation, which further impairs circulation.

It is a vicious cycle of one system slowing down the other, and the cycle spirals downward into a more severe migraine. Drainage and movement of the lymph system is extremely important to your health, including controlling migraines.

LIVER HEALTH AND YOUR EMOTIONS

Asian countries suffer from fewer migraines by percentage, and treatments are often successful without pharmaceuticals. Chinese medicine practitioners treat headaches and migraines by addressing emotional, physical, and dietary causes, and I adopted this approach on my own healing journey and found it to be effective.

Acupuncture and liver-cleansing treatments for migraines and headaches are popular in Eastern cultures and are effective for many patients. In general, the livers of people in Asian countries are also less taxed than those in Western cultures because they use more natural herbs rather than purified chemical drugs. Many Eastern cultures also drink less alcohol than Western cultures, which significantly affects liver health.

Eastern medicine also considers the impact of emotions on the health of an organ. Repressed, toxic emotions can cause health issues. In Eastern protocols, the emotions of anger, anxiety, and depression are considered when evaluating liver health. Anger in particular has long been associated with the liver.

Anger

In Western cultures, we don't recognize the correlation between anger and liver health because Western medicine doesn't address how emotions play a role in the body's health.

In fact, how you think and feel has a great impact on your health, including each organ. Having a healthy way to express emotions and not judge how you feel is very helpful in staying well.

Emotional overeating is often the result of a reaction to anger and resentment. Many people use food to comfort and soothe their troubled minds.

It is healthy to express your anger in a reasonable way; talk about how you feel or write it down. It may help to write a letter to the person you are angry with, explaining your feelings. If that person has passed away, you can still write the letter and take it to the burying place, read it, and then burn it!

It is beneficial to look constructively at why you are angry. With whom are you upset? Friends, family, strangers, spouse. Are you angry at yourself for something? Often you may react to someone else when it is your own emotional reactions that stand in the way of emotional maturity.

Discovering repressed anger is not easy. Repressed often means it is hidden and difficult to access. Seeking professional help may be necessary to heal buried emotions.

Diana's story: If you doubt the importance of emotions in improving your health, understand that I did too. In fact, it wasn't until I had hit a plateau in my healing journey that I stepped back to look at myself.

I couldn't eliminate my migraines completely until I was able to reframe my understanding of the car accident that damaged my neck and head as a teenager. I had to remove the blame I placed on the driver of the car. I had to decide to acknowledge that it was an accident. I had to forgive. When I could genuinely accept that new perspective on my events, I experienced a new level of healing my migraine pain.

WHAT TO DO NEXT

Regardless of what has overtaxed your liver, be it drugs, alcohol, emotions, environmental toxins, or other causes, getting the liver to heal and work properly is the only way to live without headaches. The nervous system needs minerals, hydration, glucose, and oxygen to function. A healthy liver protects the brain by ensuring these nutrients are readily available to your brain. How to heal the liver is discussed in **Protocol 1**.

If you have migraines, the most logical and important place to start is with the health of your liver. Your liver has tremendous regenerative powers and once you heal your liver, you should be able to eat trigger foods in moderation without a problem.

Head trauma does not need to be severe to cause neck issues and headaches.

2

Head and Neck Injuries Increase Your Risk for Migraines

Head and neck injuries are closely associated with headache pain, including migraines. Neck injuries can cause obstructions or impingements to blood vessels and spinal fluid flow, and misalignment of the cervical vertebrae (especially C1 and C2) is often involved.

Misalignments of the C1 and C2 vertebrae are generally caused by an injury to the neck or back, or a strong blow to the head. Neck or head injury, whiplash, or a concussion are common factors among migraine sufferers. According to an article on Migraine.com, head injuries are associated with migraine headaches, citing a Norwegian study that followed 105 people who had head injuries for 22 years. After 22 years, 82 percent of the women and 70 percent of the men complained of regular head pain. There is still a lot for us to learn about why head injuries cause head pain, but many people find some relief once the neck is properly aligned.

If you scored 80 or higher in the H column, this chapter applies to you. Misalignment of the upper spine is generally recognized as a contributing factor in headaches and migraines. It is possible to get migraines from head and neck injuries and misalignments without any other contributing factor.

WHY DOES NECK MISALIGNMENT AFFECT HEAD PAIN?

It is generally understood that muscle tension and neck pain can cause or exacerbate head pain. What usually isn't discussed with the patient is the reason why neck misalignment contributes to a headache.

The causes are from two issues: impeded flow of blood, nerve signals, and/or cerebrospinal fluid (CSF) around the brain and spine,[2] and the body's stress response to experiencing pinching or impingement of a vertebral artery or nerve. A small interruption in flow will not impact a heathy person as their body can adjust. For someone with low flow condition, they are not able to adjust to this reduction in flow to the head because their system is in a delicate balance with already-low resources available.

Skull Alignment

When there is pressure on the skull from misalignment (or the 22 bones of the skull have become misaligned from head injuries), just wearing a hat with slight pressure can cause a migraine. Pressure on the skull can cause pain that encompasses the entire head and creates a "squeezing" feeling. If hats cause a headache or migraine, it is likely that you have abnormal pressure on your skull from misalignment.

Impeded Flow

Arteries, veins, and a bundle of nerves pass through and around the spine, providing blood and nerve impulses to and from the brain, eyes, sinuses, ears, etc. Most people who have cervical vertebrae C1 and C2 out of alignment will experience migraine headaches or some kind of head pain—on occasion or frequently. Misalignment and/or very tight muscles can cause bones in the head, jaw, and neck to put pressure on the skull and/or pinch the vertebral nerves and blood vessels that wind through the openings in the upper vertebrae. This impedes blood and nerve flow to the head. In other words, it can cause restricted blood and oxygen delivery to the brain, as well as restricted CSF flow.

Stress Response

Additionally, when a vertebral artery or nerve is just slightly pinched, the autonomic nervous system can react to it as a threat and go into the fight-or-flight response, which further directs resources away from the brain. You may be unaware that this is happening. If muscle tension is present, it can also restrict blood flow and further complicate the issue, including impeding spinal fluid from moving up and down the spine and around the brain, which can cause the head to hurt.

There are specific practitioners who can help with these alignments. Make it a priority to find a good *craniosacral therapist* or *soft tissue manipulation* expert. This type of adjustment reduced my pain level significantly and allowed me to wear a hat without getting a headache. A list of specific certifications to look for in a practitioner is included later in this chapter.

DIFFERENT TYPES OF NECK INJURIES CAUSE HEAD PAIN

When the brain is not getting what it needs to function, it will expand the blood vessels to increase blood delivery. This causes head pain. If the brain doesn't get enough blood quickly, it will begin to shut down systems to preserve energy. That is why migraine sufferers must lie down in a dark room; they need to preserve the energy the system requires. This is a survival mechanism to prioritize blood to the brain, because if the brain stops working, the whole body could die. While this is unlikely to occur due to a migraine, the body's survival mechanism works to protect the brain.

Head trauma does not need to be severe to cause neck issues and headaches. Over time, certain muscles compensate for the misalignment, and other muscles grow weak. Long-term misalignment can cause scarring and problems that are difficult to heal.

Brain stem damage from whiplash was recently discovered to be a potential cause of pain to the ears, sinuses, face, and head. Current medical equipment and tests are insufficient to measure the immediate and long-term damage from head and neck trauma. Bruising of the brain from a concussion often leaves the brain more susceptible to future pain, possibly due to brain stem damage and other complications we are not medically aware of.

Forward Neck Syndrome

Neck and back injury are not the only cause of misalignment. *Forward neck syndrome* is becoming more prevalent today due to our near-constant use of computers and cell phones. It is a serious problem and growing worse as our dependence on technology increases. Over time, this can cause enough misalignment in the neck to reduce blood supply to the head and cause pinched nerves. Neck muscles can also grow tight and reduce blood flow through muscles. Forward neck syndrome results from long-term poor posture and can permanently realign the spine.

Desk Job Immobility

If you sit most of the day, this immobility can cause strain to the muscles of the spine, tightening the low back muscles. This tightness will creep up, vertebrae by vertebrae, and impede blood and spinal fluid flow to the head. Additionally, when you sit all day, breathing becomes shallow—and spinal fluid moves with the breath. The act of breathing is designed to slightly undulate the spine as the body flexes during inhalation and exhalation, pumping valuable spinal fluid up and down.

Sitting for long periods not only tightens the muscles, it also reduces breathing and spinal fluid motion, thereby limiting nutrients to the head.

If you are reaching in front of you all day at a desk or other job, you may be overstretching your upper back muscles and shortening your pectoral muscles, causing further tightness. Sitting also shortens your anterior (front) hip flexors and stretches your posterior (back) hip flexors, which can lead to posture problems. Shortened hip flexors, along with glut muscles not firing properly, overwork the hamstrings, causing them to lengthen and become very tight. This causes a ripple effect in the body, which can lead to tightness of all the muscles on the backside of your body, from your heels to the top of your head.

Tensing the Jaw

Jaw tightness causes migraines because the tension produces swelling in the joint and tightness in the muscles at the back of the head—and both restrict blood and nerve flow to the brain. Studies suggest TMJ (temporomandibular joint) disorders are very frequently present along with cervical vertebrae pain and migraine headaches. If you have tenderness directly below your ears and/or tight jaw muscles, it is likely that your jaw alignment and jaw tightness is related to your neck alignment and head pain.

Common Causes of TMJ Disorders

1. Injury to the jaw or neck (e.g., a blow to the face or whiplash): This is one of the most frequent causes of sudden onset or severe pain in the jaw and base of the skull at the back of the head.

2. Grinding or clenching your teeth (also called bruxism).

3. Sleep disordered breathing occurring when your airway collapses while you're asleep, blocking your breathing. The lower jaw instinctively will clamp down or thrust forward in an attempt to open the airway.

4. Arthritis can occur in any joint, including the TMJ.

5. Dislocation or erosion of the joint.

6. Improper bite alignment.

7. Poorly done dental work, such as high crowns or fillings that change how your teeth come together.

8. Tension and stress, which causes the jaw to tighten as an auto-response; this is very common among migraine sufferers.

Possible TMJ Symptoms

*   Pain and tenderness around jaw, cheeks, ears, below the ears, and neck

*   Tinnitus

*   Jaw pain or stiffness

*   Popping, grating, or clicking jaw

*   Earache

*   Inability to open jaw completely, locking jaws

*   Painful chewing

*   Tired feeling in face

*   Change of facial expression

A change in how your lower and upper teeth fit together, e.g., one side of your bite or the other doesn't meet

Jaw problems are such a common factor with those who have migraines that this area should not be overlooked. A tight jaw can be the sole cause of migraines, although it is more likely in combination with other issues. For many people, it is a dentistry problem or a misalignment and must be dealt with professionally. Jaw tightness is addressed in **Protocol 2**.

NECK, SHOULDER, AND BACK PAIN ASSOCIATED WITH MIGRAINE

If you have neck, shoulder, or back pain, and you have migraines, there are a number of specialists to assist you. I highly recommend going to see one or more of these specialists:

- Osteopath

- Chiropractor

- Doctor of Physical Therapy (DPT)

- Physical therapist with additional training: Orthopedic Certified Specialist (OCS)

- Physical therapist with this specialty: Fellow of Applied Functional Science (FAFS), Gray Institute

In addition to the upper cervical vertebrae impinging on the flow of nerve signals, spinal fluid, and blood, the upper back muscles can also affect both. In studies, the trapezius muscle of the upper/mid back has been shown to cause head pain when the lower section of this muscle is weak.[3]

See the diagram below of this muscle to help you know its location. See my online videos demonstrating exercises to strengthen this area, which have been shown to take pressure off the upper section of this muscle and allow for better blood flow to the brain. If this muscle is weak in the lower area, the upper area works too hard and causes excessive tightness, which impacts the blood flow.

WHAT ARE TRIGGER POINTS?

You may notice places on your upper back, shoulders, and neck that are painful and feel like a muscle knot. There is no actual knot, but it feels like it. These places are called trigger points and they can add to the causes of migraines.

Trigger points are tiny muscle spasms in part of the muscle. These often occur when a person is using back muscles for a repetitive task and circulation is reduced. In theory, that small patch of muscle becomes tight and chokes off its own blood supply, which irritates it even more and causes it to tighten more—and a vicious cycle called a "metabolic crisis" ensues. As a result, other muscles in the back work on behalf of the tight muscle, causing fatigue in those muscles to "creep" up the back. As more and more muscles get tight, less and less oxygen and blood are flowing steadily to the brain.

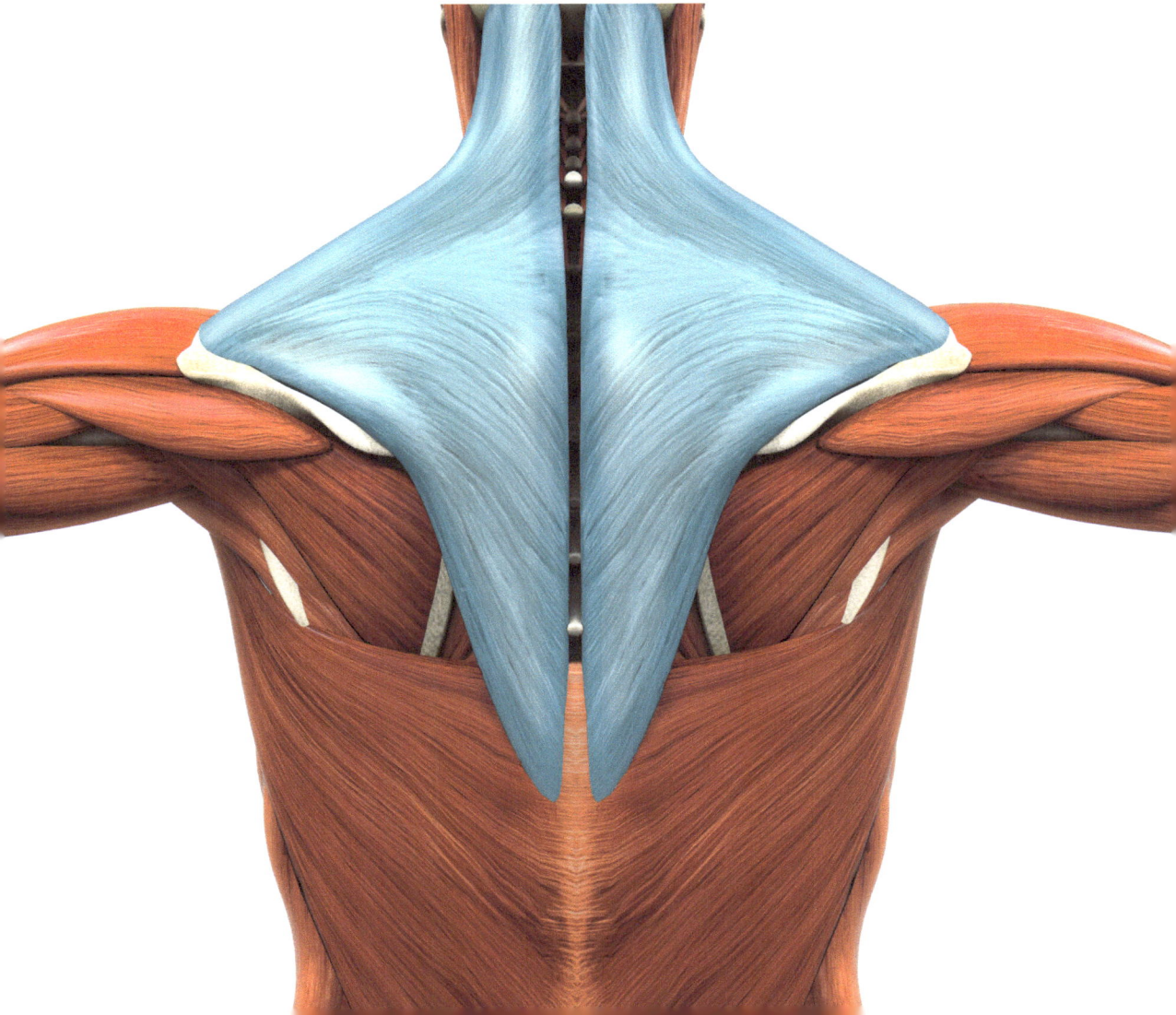

This can happen just from sitting at the computer. Your arms are forward, stretching the back for an extended period. Without movement, stretching, and good circulation, those muscles will lack oxygen and can tighten up, creating trigger points.

If the lower trapezius muscle is weak, certain activities can cause the muscle to create small spasms or trigger points. Low back injuries can have the same impact. As the low back muscles fail to do their job, other back muscles take up the slack, causing tension, fatigue, and muscle spasm. This restricts blood flow, which is a big deal when the delicate balance of blood to the head is already an issue.

> ***Diana's Story:*** *After 35 years of chiropractic care, my neck and low back are still weak. I still need to be consistent with my physical therapy exercises, which have helped tremendously when I do them. However, now that I know that low oxygen is the cause of the tight muscles, as soon as I notice it, I begin to reverse it to prevent pain with deep, slow breathing. I can change my posture, relax my jaw, stretch my neck, drink water, wiggle my spine and jaw, and breathe to feel better in moments. If I do nothing to mitigate it, it can quickly get worse. I did this as part of my* Stop, Drop, Roll, and Smile *method when I was still experiencing migraines.*

MEDICAL IMAGING

Some Western medical practitioners have recognized that the expansion of blood vessels in the brains of migraine patients is the autonomic systems' attempt to increase blood and oxygen flow to the head. Some of the medical community will say that if the cerebral blood flow was compromised, they could see that on an MRI. That is not accurate.

The medical community is working on new MRI technology that can measure blood flow in the brain in greater detail to aid in diagnosing many diseases. These include dynamic susceptibility contrast (DSC) perfusion MRI, functional MRI (fMRI), and arterial spin labeling (ASL) perfusion MRI. However, today's technology is not comprehensive or sensitive enough to detect small changes in the amount of oxygen the brain is receiving. With a migraine, the lack of supply is not as significant as with a stroke or brain injury, so it is much harder to detect through medical imagery.

Functional MRI is able to tell which area of the brain blood is flowing to, but it cannot determine if the brain is getting enough oxygen into the cells or if the magnesium supply is sufficient to allow the proper flow of fluid in and out of the cells.

In some cases, the brain will have an accumulation of blood or lymph in an area with inflammation, which does not allow good drainage. This results in increased pressure and may also cause pain. The current tests are simply not sensitive enough to detect low blood flow variation or backed-up lymph, even while headaches are occurring.

WHAT TO DO NEXT

Protocol 2 addresses spine and nervous system health. Use that information to eliminate your migraines and improve your health.

Tension hides in
many forms.

3

Stress Plays a Role in Pain

The first step in eliminating migraines caused by stress and tension is learning to be aware of your body's state—and finding ways to relax and to tell your body there is no emergency.

In today's busy and demanding world, the pressures of work, kids, home, and social life can cause enough stress to put your body into a sympathetic state ("fight or flight"). Pressure might be the only threat, but your body can respond as if a lion is chasing you. You may not be aware that this is happening.

If you scored 80 or above in the S column, this chapter is here to help.

HOW DOES STRESS CAUSE MIGRAINES?

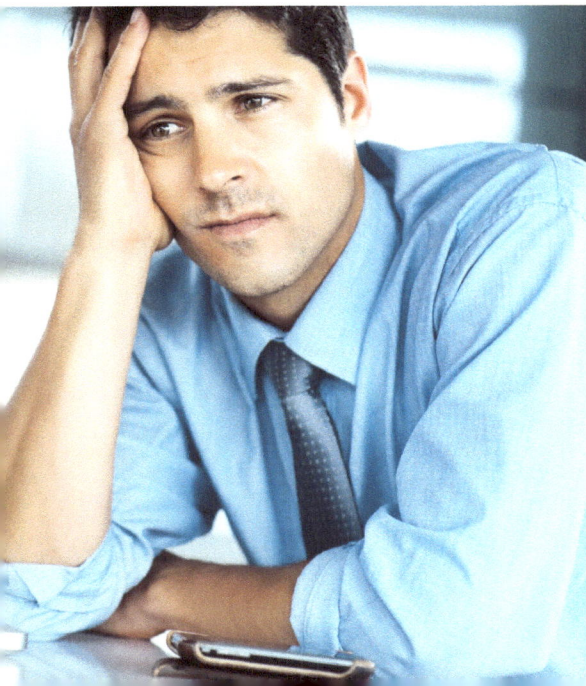

The sympathetic state is the fight-or-flight response of the nervous system, where the body prepares for a race, a fight, to flee from a wild dog, to rush to get to work on time and catch the train, or to meet a deadline at work. This response redirects oxygen, blood, and fluid away from the brain and toward other organs and muscles. It is like punching the gas pedal in your car. It will get you somewhere quickly, but it uses up a lot of fuel. Staying in the sympathetic, fight-or-flight state for long periods of time will deplete your system of resources.

One of the most valuable things I learned about migraines during my research and healing is that all migraines occur when the body is in fight-or-flight mode—and it's likely that the migraine develops because it's been in that mode too long.

MENTAL TENSION—IT'S ALL IN YOUR HEAD

No one likes to be told that stress is causing headaches. I didn't want to hear that and I didn't believe it. I meditated. I did yoga. I was conscious and aware. The last thing I wanted to believe was that my own lack of controlled relaxation was causing me to suffer. When it was pointed out to me, I denied it. I even felt resentment toward the friend who pointed it out. However, I came to learn it was true. I was one of the people who was addicted to dopamine rushes and had to get lots of work done and put heavy demands on myself. In order to heal, I had no choice but to learn to manage this stress.

When the Truth Hurts (and Helps)

Self-imposed demands can create headaches. When you are experiencing mental stress, the nervous system can go into fight or flight and this demands extra physical energy. To accommodate this need, your body will flush out calcium and magnesium through the kidneys because these two minerals relax the muscles. You don't want relaxed muscles during a real crisis. However, when the emergency is a mental struggle, the last thing you need is tense neck and shoulder muscles. Flushing out these minerals can increase muscle tension and reduce blood flow to the head.

Diana's story: A close friend once told me I was creating my migraines with my thoughts and resistance to what was happening in my life. I was defensive and angry when she said this.

I knew I was not consciously creating my head pain. I wanted the pain to stop for good. How could I possibly be creating it? But once I opened my mind a tiny crack to the possibility that I was responsible for the pain, I wondered if I could fix it.

When I realized that not only were my liver and blood vessels impacting my head pain, but so were my thoughts, I became more empowered to transform my health. Once I stopped blaming the car accident that injured my neck, working while sitting at the computer all day, and putting pressure on myself with work, I started to see how I was creating my own tension. I was making choices to push myself, putting demands on myself that I believed were critical. I was the one not breathing deeply, not relaxing, and not helping my liver to be strong so my body could function properly. I was the one taking a pill for a headache rather than a break to relax. No one else had any control over my body or my health. It was all me.

Sometimes people are not honest with themselves or they deny uncomfortable truths. Besides the possibility that our own choices and goals may be creating chronic stress, headaches can become an excuse as to why we can't go to a job we hate, why we can't join family events we don't enjoy, or why we don't have the energy to do certain tasks. We may have gotten used to saying, "No, I can't go to these activities because it will give me a headache."

Take a few moments to look closely at what advantages you might gain from your head pain. Do you get days off work that you wish you had without headaches? Do you get sympathy from your partner, children, or friends? Do you get quiet time alone that you need? Do you need more rest but never take it until it is forced upon you by a migraine? If your illness is serving you in some way and you aren't finding another way to make these things happen without the headaches, then headaches might continue in order to grant you something that you desire.

Headaches can become a scapegoat or a sort of "easy out" when you might not want to make decisions, let people down, or make commitments. You might not realize this is contributing to the tension in your body.

Headaches are the worst way to get out of doing things you don't want to— and you may not realize that's what is happening. It is less painful to disappoint someone than it is to have a three-day migraine. Decide that facing other people's emotions (or your own) is something you *can* do and are *willing* to do. Whatever it might be, if you have a reason to be ill, then it will be far more difficult to get well and find your new normal, especially if you don't fully understand what is causing it.

This is not an easy subject for people to look at. No one wants to believe they are preventing themselves from being well, but it can happen. Take a careful look at this area of your belief system. Are there any benefits to not being well? This may not apply to you, but if this was the one thing preventing you from getting completely well, isn't it worth looking at?

> *Diana's story: Eventually, I saw that tension was my choice. I could decide how I breathed, how I responded to demands, how I ate, how much fresh air I got each day, how much I stretched my neck and spine, how long I sat immobile at the computer, and how I replaced the minerals I lost due to stress. I had control over all of that, and initially I didn't realize that it affected how my head felt.*
>
> *As soon as I realized I caused tension with my thoughts and beliefs and no one but me could fix it, I knew that I had all of the power within myself to change it. This was like a door opening to a new life.*

RELEASING STRESS AND TENSION

Tension hides in many forms. Pressure at work, deadlines, unfriendly coworkers, money concerns, and poor air quality can all have the same effect. Bad lighting, a noisy environment, or repetitive movements can burden the body physically. High demands to the brain and body cause an increased need for oxygen, glucose, minerals, and hydration. This constant stimulation taxes the nervous system and can wear you out, causing exhaustion that you may often push through in order to get things done or meet the demands of your job and home life.

Emotional stress can also cause muscle tension, which can lead to headaches. You must address both the emotional component and the resulting physical component in order to relax.

Relaxation Can Take Time

A common problem with muscle tension is that is doesn't release instantly. Tension builds up gradually over time and it can take a nearly equal amount of time to unwind the tense muscles and relax completely. Allow yourself plenty of time to unwind from worry, daily stress, work issues, rushing, or physical issues that create tension.

A sedentary job spent sitting at a desk creates additional physical demands. Sitting all day has been likened to how smoking hurts the body. If you have a sedentary job, get up and move often. Do stretches regularly that help your upper back and chest muscles relax.

Once you know you have control over your blood flow, stress level, and pain because you can deliberately relax your own muscles, you will shift your patterns to prevent the problems from getting to the point of creating a headache. Eventually you will learn to reduce your tension with ease and eliminate it even during a migraine. **Protocol 3** explains how to do this.

The Role of the Fascia in Muscle Tension

Every muscle in your body is held in place by your *fascia* (an interconnected web of connective tissue that interfaces with your muscles and organs and cells, storing water and fat tissue and providing a pathway for lymph, nerves, and blood vessels). Because the fascia and the muscles are an intertwined structure throughout your body, you will never have muscle tension without fascia tension as well. They go hand in hand, and relaxing the fascia is critical to releasing muscle tension. Stretching slowly is the most effective way to release fascia *and* muscle tension, along with total body relaxation and excellent hydration. The fascia holds water like a sponge. Tight fascia and dehydration also go hand in hand.

Breathing Is Communicating With Your Body

Studies have revealed that alerting the sympathetic nervous system to take control could be as simple as holding your breath while you wait for an electronic screen to load.[4] It makes sense that creating new breathing habits and taking note of your breathing regularly could reduce your stress.

How you breathe affects your headaches. It affects your nervous system and where resources are directed in your body, and it can make your autonomic nervous system go into fight-or-flight mode. You can also deliberately control your breathing to tell your body there is no emergency, that it can relax.

Oxygen is not distributed throughout your body in the same manner, moment to moment. You have enough blood in your body to send blood cells carrying oxygen to only about one-third of your body at a time. Your body knows where to prioritize blood at any one given moment. It can instantly change that flow, depending on an injury, a sudden change in activity, an emergency, or relaxation. Blood will go where it is needed the most. Also, blood will flow where you place your attention.

Each time blood is pumped around your body by the efforts of the heart, the autonomic nervous system prioritizes where that blood is delivered. After several pumps from the heart, every area of the body has received oxygen and nutrients and then the cycle begins again, providing blood supply to the areas of the body requiring the blood the most.

Pressure or worry can easily cause a lack of sufficient oxygen to the brain due to many factors. When the body is in a state of flight or flight, up to 400 times more than normal amounts of oxygen can be directed to the muscles. This depletes resources to the brain. If the body stays in a stress response for a long time, the brain is not getting what it needs. Once the brain is not getting enough oxygen, it will expand the blood vessels in the brain to promote more blood flow. This can cause a headache or migraine and forces the body to rest in order to protect the brain, conserve resources, and direct the resources you have to the nervous system.

> ## A lack of deep breathing is one of several potential causes of low oxygen in the blood.

For most people, how you are breathing should be considered first. It is critical to breathe correctly to be headache-free and healthy.

Two Basic Breathing Patterns

Humans and animals have two basic breathing patterns. Breathing is generally controlled or influenced by the autonomic nervous system, which has two unique states: fight or flight and rest and digest.

During fight or flight, breathing is quicker, shallower, and brings air into the upper half of the lungs. It keeps the body on guard and causes cortisol, a stress hormone, to be released. Over time, continual cortisol release and staying in flight-or-flight mode will damage your health. Your brain does not get enough oxygen for normal *or* optimal functioning in this state.

Have you ever noticed that when you are really stressed, it is difficult to focus and think straight? Less oxygen and resources flow to the brain during fight-or-flight mode, making it unable to complete normal thought processes.

In the stressed mode, your body cannot rest and rejuvenate. A state of chronic rushing or pressure has many health consequences. This pattern may be so constant you don't even know you are in it.

How to Tell Your Body to Relax Through Breathing

The parasympathetic nervous system is activated by breathing into your lower lungs, using your diaphragm correctly for deep belly breathing—slow inhales and exhales. It often works best if you exhale for longer than you inhale; three seconds on the inhale, six seconds on the exhale. When you breathe in this manner, the *vagus nerve*—the longest of the 12 cranial nerve pairs, connecting the neck, heart, lungs, and abdomen to the brain—responds by telling the body all is well, so it can provide oxygen to the restorative areas of the body, including the brain.

This is the basis of the deep breathing technique that I describe in more detail in Section Two, the protocol section.

If Tension Is Your Normal

A certain level of muscle tension and pain is something the body can memorize as the norm. If you are regularly using the wrong muscles for tasks because some muscles are weak or your posture is poor, your muscles may have memorized being tight. Ongoing stress can also cause permanent muscle tension. This makes relaxing them difficult.

Unfortunately for many of us, tension can be addictive. Dopamine is a neurotransmitter that gives a feeling of pleasure. The body is rewarded with dopamine when you accomplish a task, have success, take a risk, win at a game, be competitive, and push yourself. None of these are bad things, in and of themselves. However, that pleasure reward can become addictive. You may start to push yourself too much and try to prove or accomplish too much. You may overachieve for the high of dopamine. This doesn't happen with everyone, but it is a common pattern for some—and it was for me.

In the search for the natural high from dopamine and adrenaline, you can cause yourself a lot of pain. The pleasure reward you may unconsciously seek can create tension in the body. On a short-term level this is not bad. However, when you become addicted, you will stay in a state of tension. You may feel there is no time to slow down and take a breather, or that life will catch up with you and you need to stay ahead of it. You don't realize you are addicted to a rush. Your brain just tells you to keep running to stay in the game, so you do it.

Not all people who are in this pattern will get migraines. It depends on where their system is weak. But everyone who gets stuck in the rush without fully taking time to relax, unwind, breathe, and rest will suffer some kind of health or wellness issue. In the case of migraines, the addiction to dopamine or adrenaline costs a lot. The addiction depletes the resources the brain needs and pain is the result.

Shifting out of this subconscious pattern is not an easy process. You will have to relearn what it feels like to be relaxed. Consider the possibility that it has been years since you were completely relaxed.

The only way out of this pattern is to find relaxing activities that also bring pleasure. Replace the dopamine high with a serotonin high. Instead of being extremely driven or feeling there are endless things that must be done, feel gratitude for all that you have. Feel grateful that you have 10 fingers and 10 toes. Feel grateful that you can walk, speak, swallow, smile, sing, kiss, love, read, learn, smell, carry on a conversation, drive a car, see colors, vote, and make decisions. Chances are you know people who don't have one or more of those wonderful privileges. Gratitude calms the nervous system, improves circulation, and allows the body to do needed repairs for better health.

THE POWER OF YOUR THOUGHTS

Sometimes stress is unavoidable. Divorce, moving, and changing jobs are considered to be some of the highest causes of stress. A long-term illness, injury, or the death of a loved one are other unavoidable stresses.

Many people contribute a great deal to their own stress with their thoughts, fears, worries, lack of self-esteem, or lack of self-care. If you don't care for yourself, you will have a more hectic life. Self-doubt causes stress, as does self-criticism. Being critical of other people, drivers on the road, family members, or coworkers causes stress. Not accepting what is happening, or resisting what is going on or what you might have to deal with can all cause stress.

If you feel negatively about something, you are resisting it. You make it bad by judging it.

Each of us has the option to choose how we view situations and people. We can decide that everything is working out as it should be, people are all unique, and they all make mistakes. We can decide that life is serving us a good dish or we can complain that life is only giving us lemons. This is a choice each of us makes.

An important step in healing from migraines is to think that you are healing and feeling better. Like the placebo effect, what you think about your health will come true. You are now armed with how to get well, so start to think it is already occurring and your cells will get the message. You will heal faster and have less pain as you think and believe it is true. The power in your mind is strong enough to cause your body to get well.

You may benefit from finding a community of people you can talk with about your life experiences, common emotions, challenges, and more—people who can support you in the lifestyle changes you are making in order to get well. This is a way to find encouragement, not pity. Avoid falling into a pattern of talking about how bad you feel. Your body obeys your words and beliefs.

WHAT TO DO NEXT

Protocol 3 addresses stress and tension and provides ways to help you relax and handle stress differently.

4

Critical Resources
Your Brain Needs

Chronic dehydration and an imbalance of minerals are huge contributors to most migraines. A diet high in toxins, while lacking pure water and mineral-rich foods, is an eating lifestyle that contributes to this problem. Lack of sufficient minerals in the brain can also be caused by a weakened liver. The liver stores needed minerals to deliver to the body and nervous system as needed, just as it stores glucose for the brain. When the liver is not doing its job properly, the brain can get very low on minerals and mineral supplements are needed until the liver recovers. Low levels of iron in the blood have been attributed to causing headaches due to less oxygen being carried in the blood. Iron assists the blood in carrying oxygen to the cells. This is one of many ways in which minerals affect the nutrient delivery to cells.

However, iron deficiency is not the most common problem. Studies show that around 40 percent of industrialized populations are deficient in magnesium, and in hospital patients it is over 50 percent.[5] Other contributors are chronic stress, lifestyle, and diet in modern societies, as well as chemicals that overtax the liver.

If you scored 80 or above in the M column, this chapter will provide you with valuable information.

HYDRATION IS KEY

To live headache-free, your central nervous system must have all the resources it requires—meaning adequate flow of cerebrospinal fluid, which carries oxygen, minerals, hydration, and glucose to your brain cells. Your nerve cells need proper hydration to enable delivery of nutrients. Your blood is not able to deliver nutrients effectively if you are dehydrated. You may think hydration is simply drinking enough water—but if your cells do not have proper mineral balance, they cannot utilize the water. Also, neurons need minerals to "fire" and communicate, and you may suffer head pain if you are working without enough minerals.

When we are stressed, the body flushes out magnesium and calcium in order to be more alert, because these minerals relax the body and muscles. When magnesium is low, it is difficult to relax and breathe calmly. If the liver doesn't have a reserve of magnesium to release after stress, a supplement will be needed. Low levels of magnesium prevent proper hydration and oxygen delivery to the brain and cause muscles to tighten, which further restricts blood flow to the head and contributes to migraines.

> You can impact your blood quality and oxygen delivery every day with proper breathing and hydrating with the correct mineral balance.

Being low on critical vitamins like D and B2 can also impact hydration, which means a healthy diet can make a difference

The modern diet is causing dehydration in people of all walks of life, including many people who do not have migraines. Chronic dehydration is a common factor that shows in many forms in addition to headaches, such as heart problems, stroke, high blood pressure, diabetes, and other health issues. Regular migraines are not something you are likely to die from, but they are a good indication that you need to change your lifestyle because your health could be at risk beyond a debilitating headache.

The modern diet and lifestyle cause dehydration in a few different ways. First, toxins in our food, soil, air, and water cause the liver to be taxed beyond its capacity to function as needed and store minerals the way it is supposed to. Secondly, inflammation from toxins makes the blood too thick to fit blood cells single file into capillaries to deliver oxygen and nutrients to cells. When blood is clogged with toxic matter, it is less efficient at carrying nutrients and too thick to deliver efficiently.

WHAT YOU EAT MATTERS

Additionally, the modern diet is often low in water, high in sodium, and high in saturated fat. The modern diet often steals water from organs and the fascia in order to process and digest dry, high-fat foods such as potato or corn chips. Dry foods require liquids in order to be processed through digestion. Imagine pouring coconut oil down the drain. How much water would you need to make sure it doesn't clog the drain? Compare that with coconut water. Your body needs a large amount of hydration to move coconut oil through your pipes, just like you would need to wash it down the drain. Alcohol, toxins, and pharmaceutical drugs are grossly dehydrating and require a significant amount of compensation to reverse the drying effects on your systems and organs. Additionally they can flush out precious minerals.

Only fresh food, high in natural minerals and water, such as fruit and vegetables, fresh juices, and coconut water, will increase your hydration signifi-

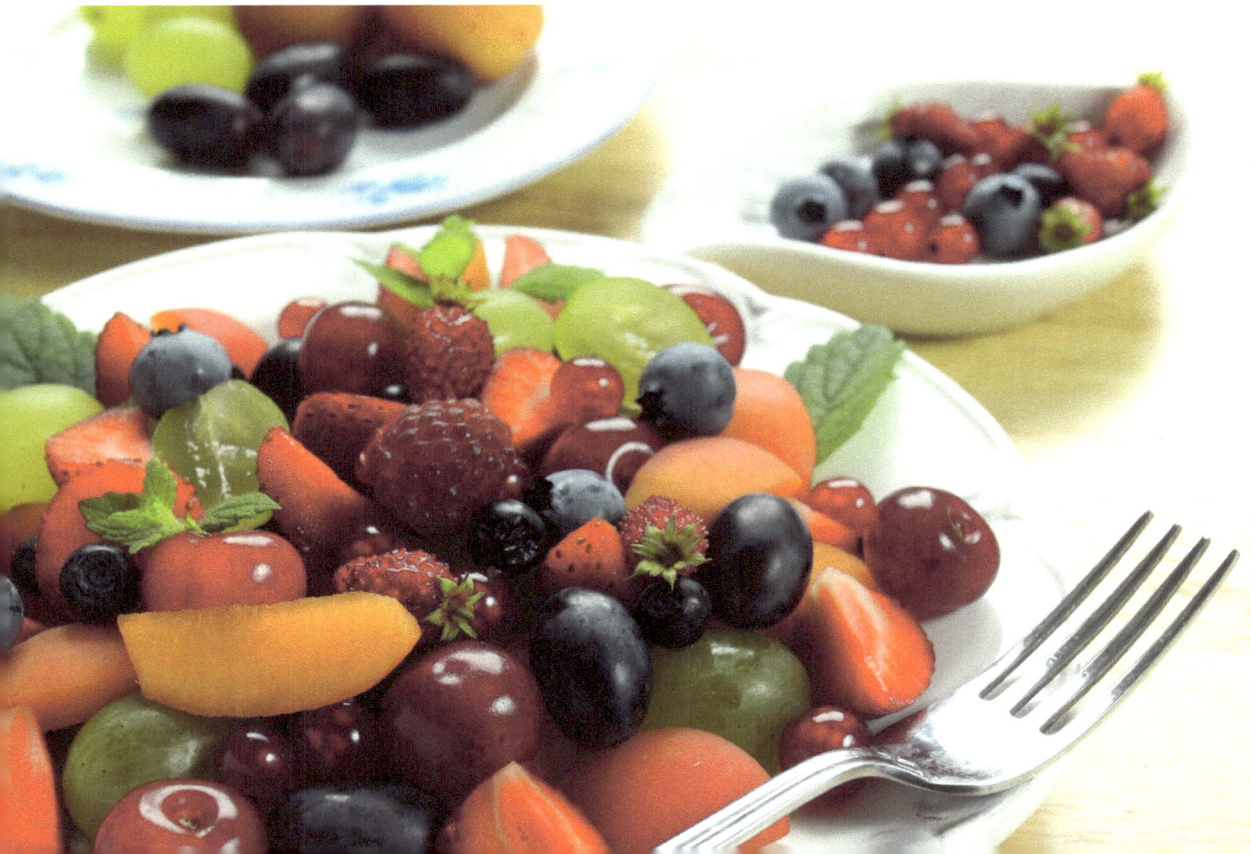

cantly. Potatoes, rice, grains, fat, animal protein, processed food, and junk food dehydrate your cells because they require a great amount of water to digest and push through your body. This is partly why doctors and nutritionists tell us to eat a diet rich in fruits and vegetables.

Many people wonder how much water they should drink. Adequate water intake depends on the situation. A widely proposed rule of thumb is that you should be drinking half of your body weight in ounces of liquids every day. This means if you weigh 150 pounds, you would need to drink 75 ounces a day. However, that is a highly generalized statement. You can definitely over-hydrate and flush critical minerals out of your body by following this rule, without making other considerations. How much water you need to drink daily varies depending on what you are eating. If you eat a diet high in fruits and vegetables and low in saturated fats, you will need far less water than a person who eats the standard American diet.

How much liquid you should drink also depends on how active you are, what you are drinking, what you are eating, and how the weather impacts your hydration. If your snacks all consist of watermelon and oranges, you will need less water than if you snack on french fries and popcorn. Fruit high in water content is hydrating, because it also contains healthy minerals and glucose. Dry foods require you to drink more, as do salty foods. If you drink tea and coffee, you need to increase your intake of water to counteract their diuretic effect.

A better rule of thumb for hydration is to monitor your output, not your intake.

If you are excreting light yellow urine throughout the day, are not going more than two hours between releasing your bladder, and you don't get even a slight headache, then you are likely drinking enough liquids. Signs that you need to increase your fluids intake are medium to dark yellow urine, sunken face, not emptying your bladder for long periods of time, fatigue, being thirsty, and slight or strong headache.

All of these factors, plus food and more, influence blood viscosity. Blood viscosity is the thickness and stickiness of blood. It is a measurement of the blood's ability to flow through the vessels, as well as how much friction the blood causes against the vessels, and how hard the heart has to work to pump your blood. Viscosity determines how much oxygen is delivered to organs and tissues. People with high blood pressure have high blood viscosity (thick blood), in part due to low hydration and toxins in the blood. High blood viscosity is easily modifiable with safe lifestyle-based interventions of food, hydration, and exercise.

Hydration is critical to the function of the blood, which is far more than a transportation system for the body's cells to receive nutrients. The blood is a very large organ. Your blood is three to four times larger by volume than your brain, and it is two to three times greater in volume than your liver. If your blood is not working right, then all of your body suffers by not receiving the oxygen and nutrients the cells need to live.

> *Diana's story:* In my late teenage years and early 20s, some days I would wake up thinking about a warm, tasty breakfast. My go-to for a while was a buttered English muffin with scrambled eggs on top, covered in melted cheese. My other standby was an open-face English muffin with peanut butter on one side and melted, dripping cheese on the other.
>
> Today, I am careful what I eat. I have to be in order to feel well. I eat small amounts of goat and sheep cheeses on rare occasion, which are far easier to digest. I may have some cheese in veggie lasagna with a salad or a protein snack without carbs. When I was still healing, cheese could still give me a headache, so I limited that. Occasionally, I was disciplined enough to eliminate it for many months at a time. Now organic cheese doesn't cause any negative effects.
>
> When I eat the right food, ample energy and feeling great are mine to enjoy. Eat the wrong foods, and the price is high, as my energy falls away and a headache or tummy ache sets in. I had no idea how great I could feel until I eliminated many foods. I didn't realize how much energy those foods were stealing from me.

WHAT TO DO NEXT

Protocol 1 addresses minerals, oxygen, and hydration. Work with your doctor, if needed, to confirm the mineral supplements you need to take, especially concerning iron. Many people do not need to supplement iron and for a small percentage, taking iron when it's not needed can be harmful. Practice moderation in adding supplements to your diet and seek out foods naturally high in minerals.

5

The Drug Connection to Migraines

Thank goodness the modern world has a pill that can eliminate severe pain in a time of crisis or after a surgery. Acute pain can quickly overwhelm a person and slow down the healing process. However, these wonder drugs that have saved us from severe suffering are often used for chronic pain, making a person's liver and body deal with the harmful effects of ingesting these drugs on a long-term basis.

Painkillers might better be labeled simply as "killers," because an American citizen dies every 15 minutes from taking prescription opiates.

If you scored higher than 80 points in the B column, please read this chapter.

BLOOD VESSELS: THE DRUG CONNECTION

Many prescription and OTC drugs damage your blood vessels, and long-term use causes damage that takes time to heal. The labels on all bottles of ibuprofen

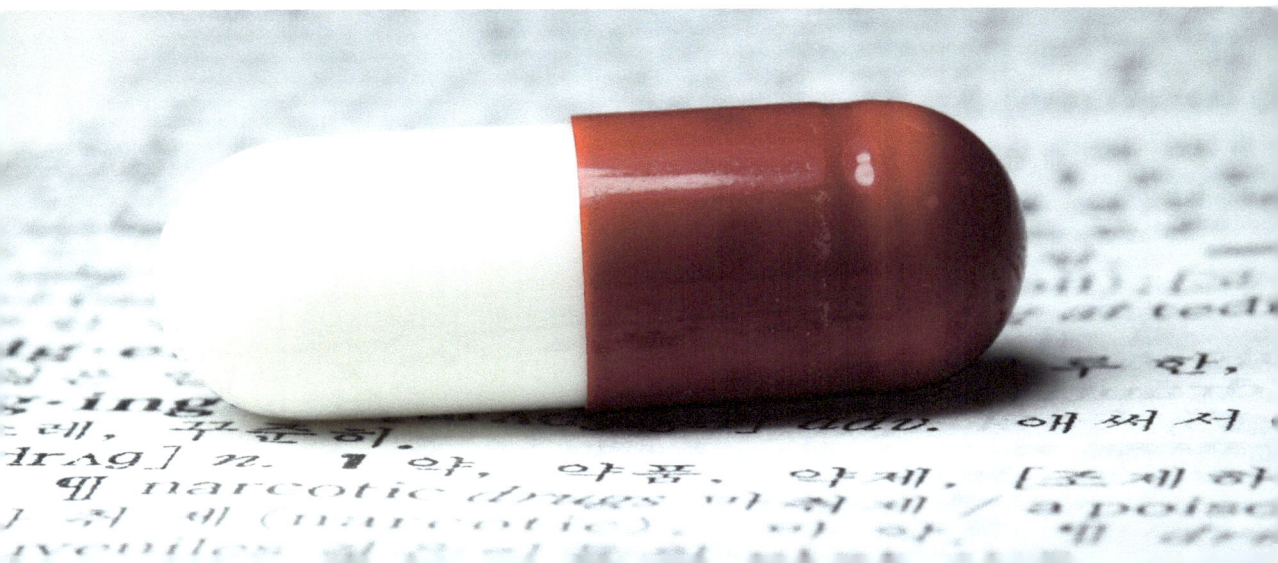

state that taking it will increase your risk of heart attack and stroke because of the harm it does to blood vessels.[6] Blood vessels have muscular walls that make them capable of expanding and contracting. Drugs that force vessels to expand or contract injure the muscle wall over time. Damaged blood vessels cannot expand and contract properly, leading to many health issues, including possibly migraines.

Blood delivers oxygen, and blood vessels deliver blood. Blood vessels consist of arteries (coming from the heart), veins (returning to the heart and delivering to the liver, kidney, and lungs), and capillaries (which connect the arteries, veins, and cells). Capillaries make delivery of nutrients to and removal of waste from the cells possible. Your body has over one billion capillaries that would cover a surface area of 1,000 square miles. If put them end to end, your blood vessels would reach 60,000 miles.[7] These tiny capillaries are an important component in getting nutrients to the cells as well as delivering back to the blood the waste to be carried away.

Blood does not enter your cells. As mentioned earlier, blood cells are like buses; they deliver nutrients and take waste away. They just go back and forth, dropping off and picking up. Blood cells carry the oxygen and nutrients that the cells need. The blood cells are pushed single file through your capillaries, where the liquid plasma in the blood cell is squeezed out through the capillary walls into the capillary bed where the cells receive it. The capillary walls do not allow certain proteins and larger things, including the blood cells, to go through the walls. All cells of the body are in close proximity to capillaries, which provide each cell with plasma.

For the capillaries to deliver what the cells require, your blood should not be too sticky, thick, or inflamed, because blood cells are larger in diameter than the capillaries. The blood cells elongate just enough to fit into the capillaries. Inflamed or sticky blood does not fit well into the small capillaries. Additionally, the proper mineral balance is essential to cause the fluid to flow in and out. Several salts are responsible for the passage of fluid through the pores of the capillary walls and for the movement of fluid into and out of each cell. All of this means that without healthy blood vessels and capillaries, nutrients and oxygen are not delivered to cells, which then cause problems and can cause headaches.

> Healthy blood vessels and capillaries that work properly are two of the most critical factors for health on many levels and especially for a pain-free head.

When the blood vessels or the capillaries are damaged and the body is facing other issues, there can be enough imbalance to prevent proper permeability of fluid into the capillary bed and into the cells, which means that cells are not nourished and hydrated. You can drink enough water and still be dehydrated if your mineral balance is off or if your blood vessels and capillaries are damaged—and this doesn't allow the nutrients to get to the cells. Over time, other diseases can develop due to this lack of oxygen and nutrient delivery.

Many migraine sufferers experience this problem. Statistics show that 72 percent of migraine sufferers have experienced a migraine triggered by a change in barometric pressure from stormy weather or an altitude change like flying in an airplane. When atmospheric pressure changes, the body should respond by changing the pressure within the body to maintain the correct flow of blood and other vital fluids. The body does this by expanding or contracting the blood vessels to compensate for the exterior change in atmospheric pressure. If the arteries cannot expand or contract as needed, due to damage to the lining of the vascular muscle wall, then not enough oxygen gets to the brain during the barometric change.

Lack of sufficient oxygen is the reason people get altitude sickness, which causes a giant migraine. Lack of oxygen to the brain is why mountain climbers die of cerebral or pulmonary edema, which is swelling of the arteries and tissues due to lack of oxygen. Mountain climbers go to mid-altitude levels and slowly acclimate to the lower amounts of oxygen in the air. While they acclimate, their bodies make more blood cells so the blood can deliver more oxygen. Making more blood cells is not enough for a person with damaged blood vessels, because more blood cells cannot deliver more oxygen if the vessels don't have the capacity to expand to deliver more blood.

> *Diana's story: I experienced symptoms during altitude changes and airplane flights, with some symptoms mimicking seizures or mild strokes. These included loss of speech, loss of fine motor skills, difficulty walking, loss of voice, and sight issues. These were all due to lack of oxygen because my blood vessels were unable to expand or contract as needed. For a couple of years, I was not able to fly in an airplane or change altitude because the symptoms were too severe. After I healed myself of migraines, those problems disappeared completely.*

Many migraine sufferers may experience milder symptoms than mine, if their blood vessels are only slightly compromised.

You don't have to be a Motrin/Advil popper for every little pain in order to have damage to your blood vessels. Diabetes and other diseases in the body can also damage the blood vessels. The health of your blood vessels is only one of the regulators that control oxygen to your cells and to your head. However, if you notice you often or occasionally get migraines from altitude changes, storms, or barometric pressure changes, or you get rebound headaches after taking medication, then you should pay attention to this chapter and consider **Protocol 1**.

Scientific studies have proven that NSAIDs (nonsteroidal anti-inflammatory drugs) and other OTC and prescription painkilling medications are some of the drugs that cause harm to blood vessels when used on a regular basis. NSAIDS include aspirin, naproxen, and ibuprofen. The OTC and prescription medications in this list include triptans, decongestants, antihistamines, and opiates such as hydrocodone, codeine, oxycodone (OxyContin, and many others),

THE DRUG CONNECTION TO MIGRAINES

Percocet (oxycodone and acetaminophen), and morphine.[8] This is stated on the warning labels for these medications as a caution that they can increase your risk of heart attack and stroke. What isn't stated is they can increase your risk of your migraines becoming more intensely painful and/or more frequent. You must safely stop all of these drugs, with the help of your doctor, if you wish to heal the damage to your blood vessels that may be contributing to your migraines.

Visit my website at RealMigraineSolutions.com for a more complete list of these medications.

Opiates are among the costliest drugs to overall body health, causing damage to the heart, lungs, brain, digestive system, nervous system, and vascular system. Opiates have a more indirect effect on the vascular system because they dull the autonomic neurological response, which controls and regulates many of the automated systems of the body. Opiates are what hospitals and hospice providers give terminal patients to help them die pain-free. With a sedative dose of an opiate, a patient will typically die in about one week, which demonstrates the harm this drug does to the body.

Diana's story: After 35 years of taking hydrocodone for my occasional migraines, it stopped working for me. In 2014, My doctor told me opiates could cause health issues and are not recommended for headaches. I am grateful to him for not allowing me to continue with this medication. He was the only doctor who told me anything negative about Vicodin, codeine, and hydrocodone, all of which had been prescribed to me for headaches for most of my adult life.

Opiate painkillers and heroin are among the most addictive drugs, and the consequences of abusing these drugs can be deadly. In 2012, the CDC estimated that 46 people die from overdoses of prescription painkillers every day in the U.S. Opiates cause the person to stop breathing. These painkillers are dangerous and should be avoided for regular use.

SYMPTOMS OF BLOOD VESSEL DAMAGE

How do you know if you have damage to your blood vessels? Migraine sufferers who have used any of these drugs and now have blood vessel damage may also notice other symptoms such as these:

- Increased heart rate when having a migraine

- Migraine headaches from incoming storms or barometric pressure changes

- Migraines caused by change in altitude (even a small amount like 1,500 ft)

- Rebound headaches from taking medications

- Lightheadedness

- Lack of focus, or speech or vision issues

- Cold hands and feet or not tolerating heat well

- Diagnosed with Raynaud's or poor circulation

It is ironically unfortunate that the drugs used to treat migraine symptoms cause more headaches, tempting sufferers to reach for more drugs. It is a vicious cycle that impairs healing. It is vital that everyone who suffers from headaches—migraine or other types—stop taking the drugs that are causing more damage. How to do that without suffering greatly will be covered in Section Two, the Protocols.

Let your medical doctor know that you want to discontinue any medications you can do without and discuss any risks associated with this. You may need to stay on some medications for other medical issues. Also discuss any herbal supplements your other practitioners prescribe to support blood vessel health, to avoid interaction issues with herbal and prescription or OTC medications. Then follow your doctor's recommendations.

Diana's story: *For 35 years, I took opiates only a few times per year. After many years of pain medication for neck pain and occasional migraines (everything from aspirin to codeine), I became deathly allergic to aspirin, suffering anaphylactic shock, and then eventually codeine stopped working and caused me to feel sick and fuzzy-headed. Suddenly, my migraines increased and I was overwhelmed by the frequency of them. I took the medications I still could more often to escape the pain, and eventually suffered rebound headaches from every dose of medication I took.*

I stopped all medications for pain management, cold turkey, when I realized they were causing more migraines. Within two weeks, I had fewer migraines simply because I no longer took triptans.

If I could do it over again, I would use the techniques described in Section Two, the Protocol section, to alleviate migraines and skip the medication altogether. Had I done this, I would have had far fewer migraines and healed much faster.

Here is a scenario to consider. Let's say that you get only a couple of migraines per year. You know they are caused by overwhelming tension and stressful situations, possibly after lack of sleep or dehydration. You don't feel that you have time to address the tension by taking a break, so you take a convenient pharmaceutical pain reliever or migraine pill, to just be done with the headache. This only happens a couple times per year so you feel that your body can handle the occasional side effects of the drug. What you're not considering is that the brain is crying out because it needs something, and the medication is covering up the symptoms generated by what the body needs.

Your body is saying, "I don't need medication. I need sleep, water, minerals, neck alignment, relaxation, a back rub, grounding, and connection with people—or more serotonin, non-inflammatory foods, or less stress. Please don't mask my symptoms with a drug. Just give me what I need."

Sleeping is very restorative to the nervous system and helps the body replenish resources. Adequate, regular sleep allows the liver to do its job of cleaning the blood and supporting the nervous system. Sometimes sleep is all that is needed to recover and that is why the brain and body force us to go to bed with a migraine. Sleeping helps restore what the nerves, brain, and body need.

The pills are convenient when stress is high and you are in the thick of it, but keep in mind they hide a problem your brain is signaling you to fix. Pain is the body's way to draw attention to a problem. The problem can be remedied without the need to cover it up. Covering it up can allow it to get worse.

Ask yourself this question: If you knew that medication taken over time would cause you to have more migraines, would you still take that pill?

If you knew that lack of oxygen to your brain caused your pain, would you take a pill and not address the lack of oxygen? Lack of oxygen can be remedied with hydration, time to calm your breathing, rest, or a number of things the body wants more than medication. The protocols I provide for living pain-free are also recipes for general well-being.

THE SAFEST DRUG

As of 2019, cannabis is fully illegal in only 10 out of the 50 states, 40 of which now recognize medical cannabis as valuable to patients[9] because it has been widely recognized as excellent for so many health needs—including relieving headaches, if you get the right kind of cannabis and take it early in the headache. Many other countries are following suit. The FDA approved the drug Epidiolex in 2018, which is CBD derived from cannabis, for the treatment of seizures. It turns out that CBD is incredibly effective with many brain disorders.[10]

Cannabis doesn't harm the blood vessels, even though it does help promote circulation and has been shown to reduce inflammation throughout the body. However, inflammation is the result of an issue in the body and not the cause of the health issue. New studies have proven that cannabinoids from the cannabis plant not only reduce inflammation throughout the body, but also work within the brain—which other medications don't do.[11] Conversely, anti-inflammatory medications are known to be unable to pass the blood-brain barrier and therefore they do not reduce inflammation in the brain.

Cannabis reduces inflammation the same way that turmeric and echinacea do, by supporting the chemistry of the body and brain on the molecular level for balance and well-being. These natural anti-inflammatories don't trick the body into reducing inflammation like medications do. Instead, they support homeostasis in the body and brain, in part by providing the brain with valuable cannabinoids that it needs.

All Vertebrates Have Cannabinoid Receptors

The brains of nearly every living animal with vertebrae have what are called cannabinoid receptors—which was discovered in 1988 first in a rat—and these receptors are part of the endocannabinoid system in humans and animals.

In a healthy person, the body naturally makes the cannabinoids. These natural cannabinoids balance the body and put it into a homeostasis state of calm and well-being. It accomplishes this by quieting hormones and neurotransmitters that excite the nervous system, and the ingested cannabinoids work the same way as the cannabinoids produced naturally by the brain. Those who study the endocannabinoid system of the body estimate that when the homeostasis of the body is thrown off, the brain stops making cannabinoids naturally, which function to reduce the impact of stress hormones. The body produces stress hormones with or without cannabinoids, but cannabinoids reduce the impact of stress hormones.

If the body is not able to make the cannabinoids, it can utilize "phytocannabinoids," other plant-derived natural products that are accepted by the body's cannabinoid receptors, from a handful of medicinal plants like turmeric, chocolate, echinacea, liverwort, grapes, tea (Camellia sinensis), brassica vegetables, and cannabis, to name a few.[12] The U.S. National Library of Medicine has a report noting that even hemp seed oil, free of the psychoactive THC, contains valuable cannabinoids that are beneficial to the brain.[13] Hemp seeds and their oil also contain valuable fat and proteins that help the brain.[14] Medical studies are showing that the body's endocannabinoid system regulates immune function, pain, and inflammation. All three of these benefits help reduce migraine pain, especially with some consistent use of the cannabis plant.

Cannabis and hemp-derived CBD oil will help your body do what the body does naturally: rest and heal. They are natural anti-inflammatories and natural relaxants. In dealing with pain and stress, medical cannabis can help your body set a new baseline for relaxation. And many of these benefits are available from hemp and hemp-derived CBD oil, which has no psychoactive component (THC, tetrahydrocannabinol). The laws in the U.S. are rapidly changing around this topic and each year it is becoming more available due to the discovery of the health benefits.

CBD oils, with low to zero THC, are proving to be very useful for certain medical needs. A patient can take CBD oil regularly without feeling "high" and it will still calm the patient's nervous system. Ingesting CBD oil is much easier on the body than smoking the plant buds. Although these buds do not produce the effect of feeling high, CBD oils with low amounts of psychoactive THC are still regulated by the federal government and are only legal in 34 states, per the date of this writing. However, for those who have legal access, CBD, as the oil or raw plant, provides cannabinoids that benefit the nervous system.

An important point is that people do not die from ingesting medical cannabis or CBD oil, but they are dying from prescription pain medication.

Doctors may hesitate to prescribe medical cannabis in states where it is legal, in part because the results can be unpredictable. However, the FDA has recently approved some CBD and THC prescription medications, which will make it easier for doctors to feel comfortable prescribing it. Doctors don't like the inconsistencies of the natural product, because there is little to no testing of doses or varieties of the plant for different conditions. Doctors may also feel more comfortable prescribing drugs that have been extensively studied. However, the states that have legalized medical cannabis did so because it is an effective treatment for many ailments and the benefits far outweigh the challenge of finding the right dosage.

Ultimately, this is a personal choice. It is still a drug. I firmly believe it is the safest of any of the pharmaceutical options. I suggest that you do your own research on this option and make the decision that is right for you.

If you can't get cannabis or don't want to use it, you will have to be more diligent with the many other means listed to address headache pain, until you are completely well. Getting well may take a year or more of healing the body. During that time, head pain will likely come and go, and should diminish over time.

Diana's Story: In the beginning, I used medical cannabis because it was the only way I could sleep at night through the overwhelming migraine pain. Eventually I used it to lower my overstimulated baseline level of stress and remind my body what it felt like to relax. Cannabis helped me find balance, homeostasis, and well-being, which is the reason our bodies are supposed to make their own.

HEALTHY MENSTRUATION FOR GOOD OXYGEN AND BLOOD FLOW

Around 50 percent of women with migraines experience their migraine pain in relation to the phases of their monthly cycle. This is caused, in part, by the hormonal changes. Levels of estrogen directly affect other hormones in the body, including serotonin—an important one for migraines. Low serotonin has many effects, including lowering healthy body functions, tightening the fascia, and slowing breathing. Lower estrogen levels can cause migraines indirectly by influencing serotonin. However, there is more to the menstruation story.

Two main factors related to menstruation impact blood flow to the brain. First, menstrual bleeding redirects the flow of blood in the body, slightly altering the flow of blood toward the womb and making slightly less available to the brain. This is not a negative factor for a woman with adequate blood flow in general and high serotonin levels. It does impact a woman with low flow condition or a low satisfaction level with her life, even if it is for only a few days per month.

When menstruation affects blood flow and certain hormones, it can increase nerve sensitivity, and this change in blood flow adds one more challenge to the already-compromised systems. A menstruating woman should increase her fluid intake, rest her nervous system, increase her slow, deep breathing, and eat foods that support excellent circulation of the blood. In general, she should rest, especially if headaches are a part of her cycle. Pleasure, joy, and gratitude need to be increased to boost her serotonin.

Second, estrogen is at its highest level around day 14 of the normal menstrual cycle. Estrogen increases blood viscosity (thickness). This can negatively impact a woman with low flow condition, especially if thick blood is already an issue. Additionally, women who are perimenopausal commonly have an irregular spike in estrogen during the month.

One of the reasons perimenopausal women have migraines is due in part to estrogen spikes affecting blood flow and serotonin. Low flow condition creates such a sensitivity that even a slight factor that impacts the delicate balance of oxygen delivery can trigger a headache. The best mitigation for these spikes is to eat blood-thinning foods (see the list in the Appendix), focus on adequate hydration, and get plenty of exercise, which also promotes thinner blood. Resting the nervous system as well as following **Protocol 1** will help to reduce or eliminate migraines.

WHAT TO DO NEXT

Protocol 1 addresses blood vessel damage and thick blood through lifestyle and dietary changes along with reducing or eliminating OTC and prescription medications.

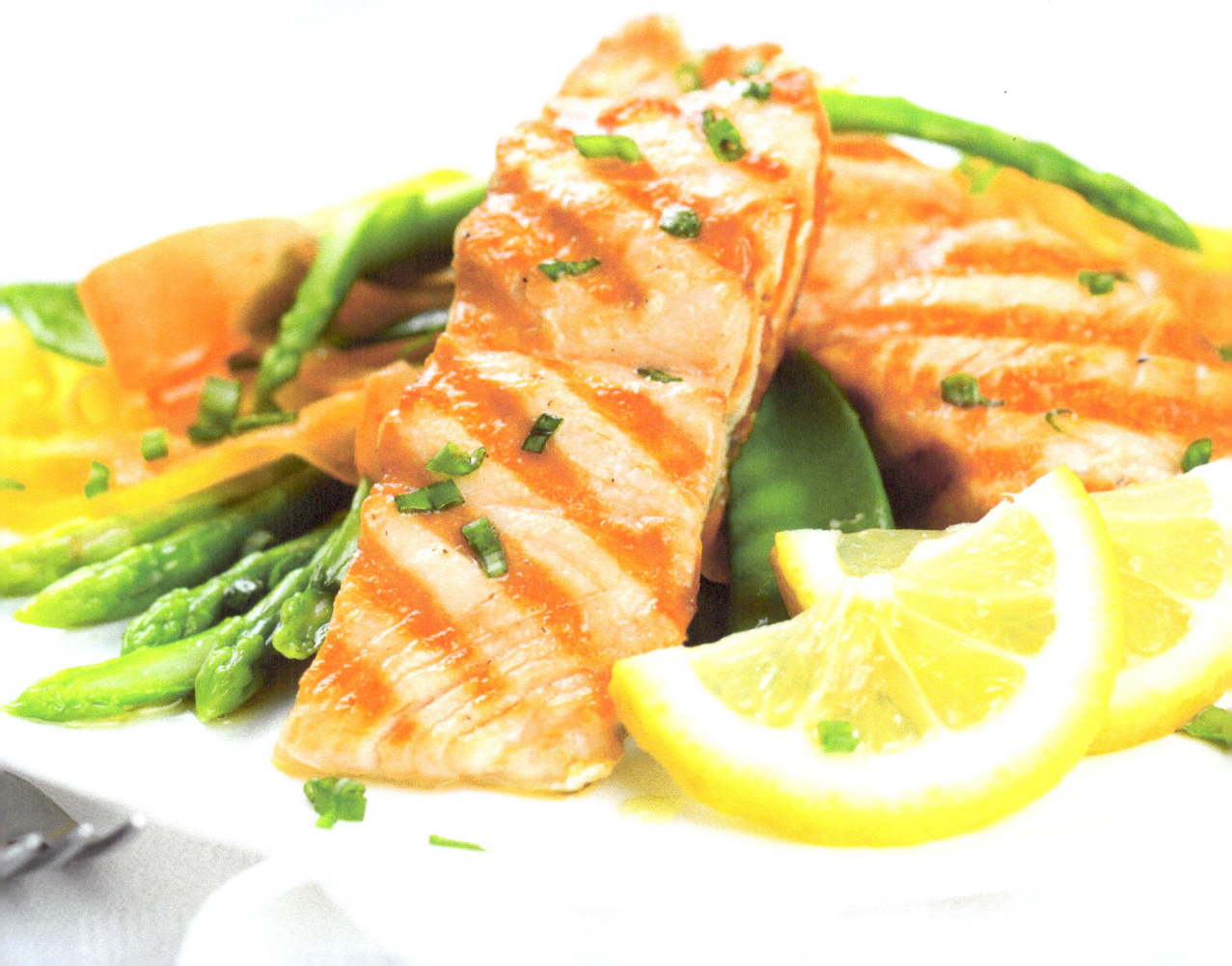

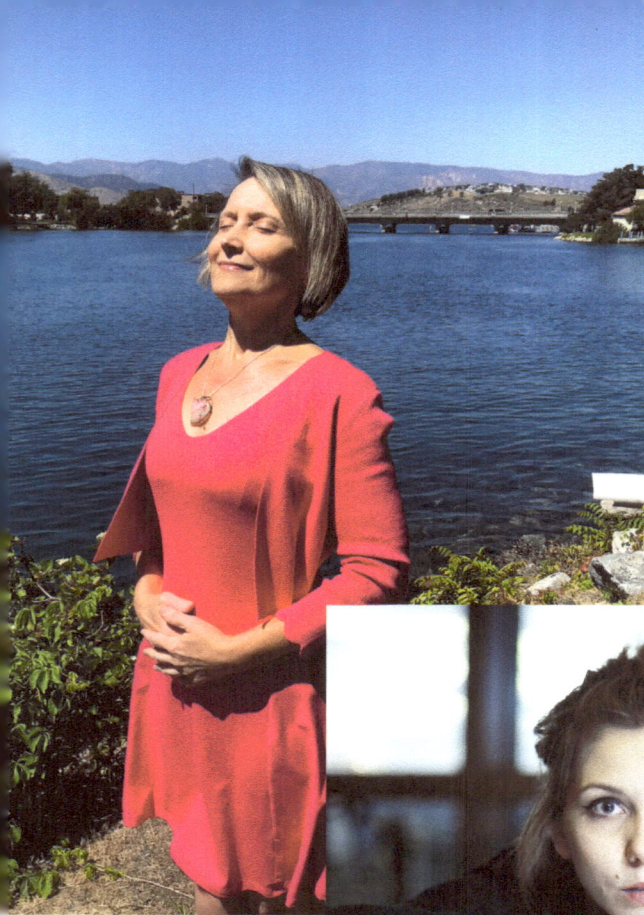

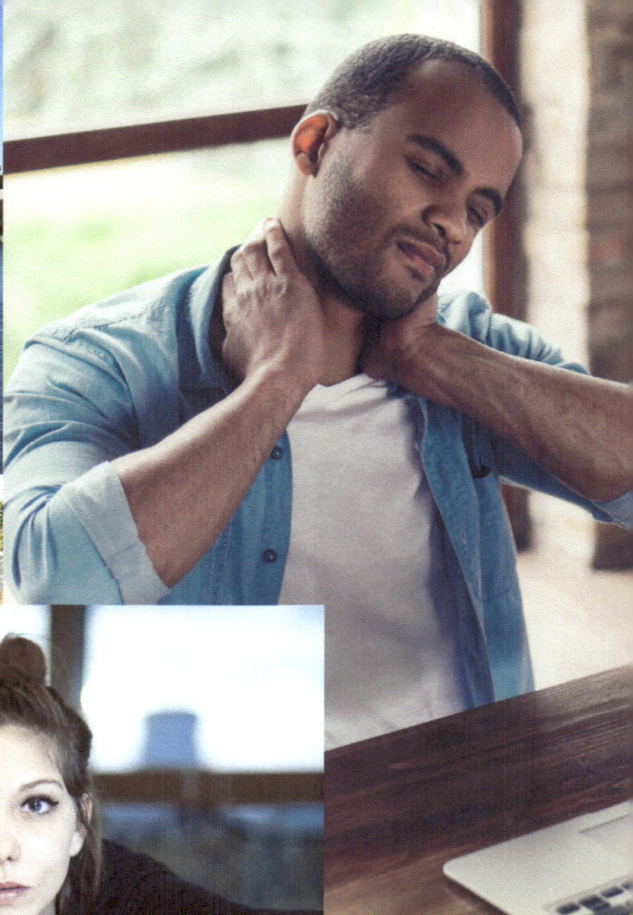

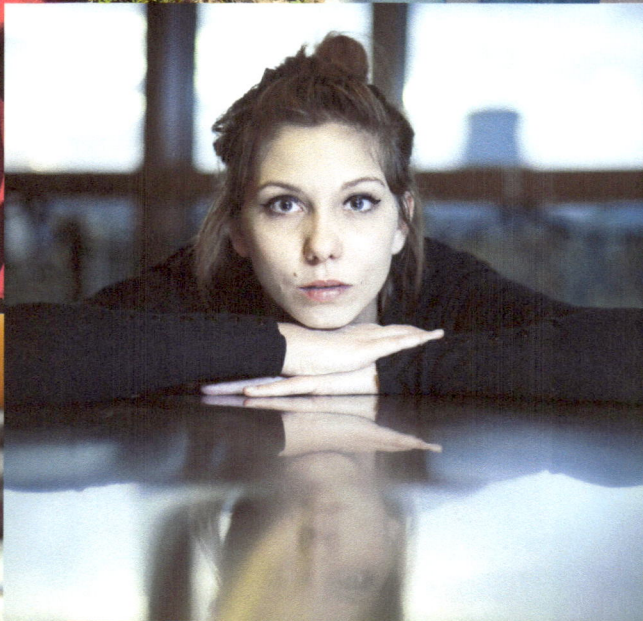

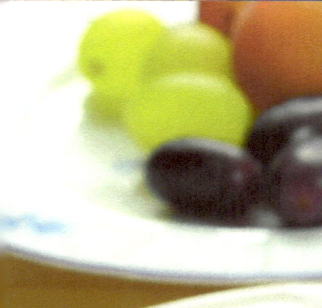

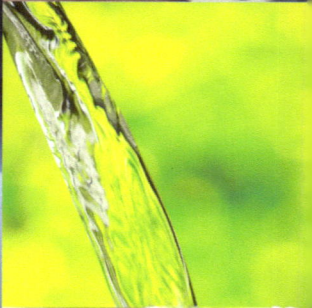

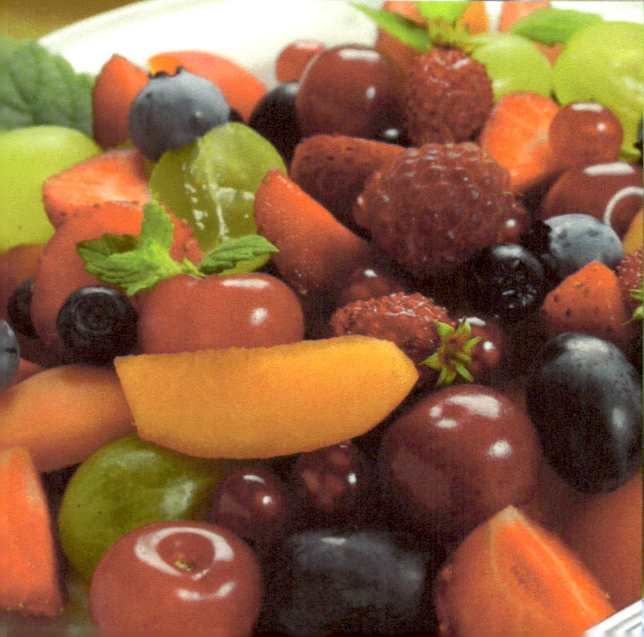

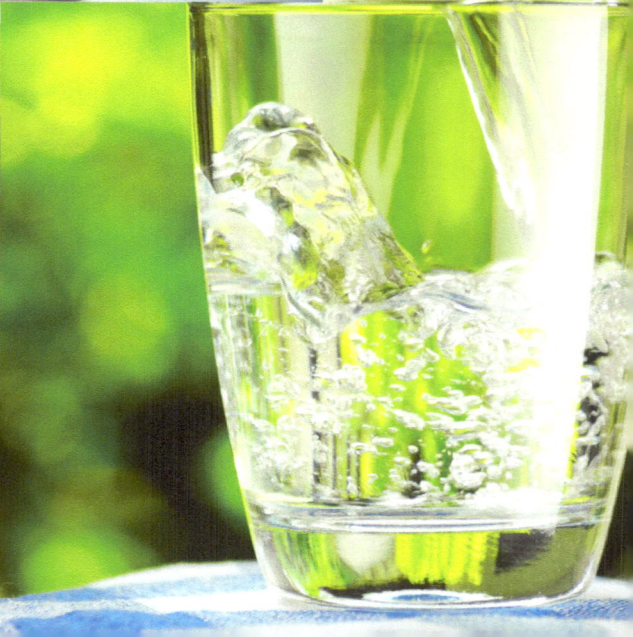

SECTION TWO

The Protocols

This section includes two methods for dealing with migraines as they are developing—the *Stop, Drop, Roll, and Smile* method and the introduction to deep breathing, which is a critical tool for every headache sufferer.

Following those, **Protocols 1**, **2**, and **3** address long-term healing solutions for the five main causes of low flow migraines. The Migraine Test early in the book helps you identify your underlying causes, which chapters to read, and which protocols you will need for healing.

The key to getting a migraine to "go away" in the short term is to **move your body out of fight-or-flight mode, prior to and during a migraine.** The migraine will not abate until you move into rest-and-digest mode—the healing state. Throughout this section, you will learn more about how to make this shift.

When you make this shift, more resources—especially oxygen—will be delivered to your brain. Although your brain needs several resources in order to avoid a migraine, none is more critical than oxygen. If you can fill your body and brain with more oxygen, a migraine will begin to dissipate.

Moving from fight or flight into rest and digest is not necessarily easy and doesn't automatically happen just because you want to do it. Something caused your body to be in fight or flight, and you can try to override the systems—sometimes without success.

The Stop, Drop, Roll, and Smile method is specifically for moving your body from fight-or-flight mode into rest-and-digest mode. This process will shift more resources from your muscles to your brain, giving it what it needs.

The deep breathing exercise is a critical tool for helping your body go into rest-and-digest mode, and making it a habit can help you prevent a migraine from starting—prevent your body from going into the fight-or-flight mode.

STOP, DROP, ROLL, AND SMILE: EMERGENCY MIGRAINE PAIN MANAGEMENT

A migraine is similar to a fire. It starts small and can quickly get out of control. When a flame is small, extinguishing it is easy. As with any blaze, once it is a raging, forest-fire-sized migraine, it takes a lot more time and resources to put out those hot flames.

Begin at the first signs to stop the fire from spreading and you will conquer it. Otherwise, it might have to burn itself out over a few days.

This method addresses temporary fixes to the underlying causes of headaches, including hydration, nutrients, and physical and emotional stress.

STOP
DROP
ROLL
SMILE

1. **STOP** what you are doing so you can be completely present with your current physical state and stop stimulating the nervous system. No phone, no computer, no TV. Provide super hydration that your brain and body need, right now. ("Super" hydration is water with natural glucose and minerals from juices or high water-content fruits such as orange juice, coconut water, celery or celery juice, or watermelon. See the Bonus Material for more details.)

2. **DROP** your breath into your belly and breathe as you expand your diaphragm with slow, calm, deep breaths. Drop your awareness into your body.

3. **ROLL** out the tension in your shoulders on a foam roller or hard surface edge, or get someone to give you 10 minutes of deep shoulder, neck, and back rubbing. You can also do any of the listed relaxation techniques (see ROLL section). Relax the jaw, drop the shoulders, and focus on calming your emotions. Move the spine to circulate the spinal fluid.

4. **SMILE** and feel gratitude to wash away cortisol. The act of smiling and feeling gratitude releases serotonin, which replaces the stress hormone cortisol. Think of things and people in your life you are thankful for.

This is so important I am saying it again: *Understand that a migraine is a cry for help from your body.* You can relieve a headache by "fixing" or satisfying the underlying causes. When you provide your body what it needs, the headaches will be greatly diminished and can go away completely. It may take an hour or more, depending on how long the migraine was developing. Migraines come on gradually and likely don't go away instantly, even though we wish they would. They gradually dissipate as the brain gets what it needs.

Stop, Drop, Roll, and Smile will help relax your body.

More details on this process can be found in my book *Stop, Drop, Roll, and Smile for Migraine Relief.*

CRITICAL TOOL: DEEP BREATHING

Breathing deep into the belly (diaphragmatic breathing), which allows the lower lungs to fill with air, is a technique that relaxes the vagus nerve and then regulates the amount of oxygen flow to the brain. Visualize your diaphragm as a tube connecting your diaphragm to your nose and imagine that tube opening and expanding to move more air, more quickly. (You don't literally have a tube from your diaphragm to your nose. It is imaginary to help you feel that connection to the breath. But the diaphragm does work like a bellows that opens and closes to draw in and express air.)

Breathing properly to stimulate the vagus nerve means expanding your diaphragm, a muscle located horizontally between the chest cavity and belly cavity. Also known as "belly breathing," diaphragmatic breathing is characterized by an expansion of the abdomen instead of the chest. To breathe in as deeply as possible, first expand your diaphragm all the way, then expand your chest to fully fill your lungs.

Do belly breathing several times per day and try to remember to breathe this way all the time. It will become more natural to breathe this way, although at first it may be a challenge. Use deep breathing exercises to make relaxation a part of every day.

Doing slow breathing while undulating the spine helps move the spinal fluid to the brain, providing more nutrients. To get fast results, overexaggerate the movement of the spine with the breath, the way it is done in *Qigong*. Qigong movements synchronize the breath with the spinal movements, pumping the fluid up and down the spinal column.

"Deep breathing" sounds simple but there is more to it than you may guess. Try these tips below and find what works for you.

Here are ways to practice deep breathing:

1. **Start with being *present*.** Close your eyes and breathe deeply for several minutes. Breathe slowly in and slowly out, as slow as you comfortably can while getting enough air. Relax your throat

so you sound like you are snoring. Next, move your awareness around your body to notice how your toes feel, how your neck feels, how your face and jaw feel. Consciously relax each muscle in your body by starting with your toes, feet, ankles, and calves. Gradually work your way up your body, but don't move on to the next body part until you have relaxed the part you are focused on. Intentionally feel a sense of calm while you do this. Know that everything is well and you are right where you need to be. Take your time. Enjoy several minutes of deep, relaxing breathing with your eyes closed, until you feel totally calm and well.

2. **Exhale longer than you inhale.** Try something like three seconds of inhale to six seconds of exhale. By fully expressing your air, you release more carbon dioxide and clean your blood, allowing for more oxygen in the body. Do the best you can. While doing this, notice that you can open your airways intentionally by thinking about it, which allows for better airflow and a quick relief from pain by opening your nostrils and your throat. This method in particular communicates to the vagus nerve that all is well.

3. **Try Qigong.** Qigong is a form of enhanced deep breathing. Practicing Qigong can be very helpful in increasing the oxygen level in your body. Qigong is an oriental practice of relaxing breath with gentle spinal movements. It is often called "yoga breathing." Essentially, any activity that makes you focus on deep breathing without strenuous exercise is effective. This is not the same as doing exercise. It is just deep breathing without using a lot of muscles because you don't want all the oxygen to be used up by the muscles. You want the oxygen for the nervous system. For more information about Qigong, see https://www.nqa.org/what-is-qigong-.

TO BEGIN THE PROTOCOLS: UNDERSTAND THE HEALING PROCESS

Healing your body from migraines is a process. Mine took me two and a half years, and now I work daily to maintain my health with exercises, meditation, and, while I am healed enough that I can eat what used to be my trigger foods, I still limit these.

Your Health Is in Your Hands

I have learned that one of the healthiest things we can do is recognize that medical doctors don't have all of the answers to how the human body works, and patients need to stop expecting doctors to fix every ailment that seizes them. As I learned this for myself, I realized that I had been considering myself a victim of my circumstances, and I could not escape my migraine pain as long as I believed that. I had to independently make my own decisions to move toward healing.

The most powerful thing we can do as individuals is understand that we are responsible for our own health—and that responsibility does not lie in the hands of our doctors. They are here to support us, educate us, and provide medication and treatment *if* necessary. The more we care for our own bodies, with consciousness placed on what we eat, how much we move our muscles, and what we think, the less we will need procedures and medications.

Listen to your body. Pay attention to the messages it delivers to the brain daily, and you will discover that in addition to the many physical contributors to migraines, there are nonphysical causes as well. Your thoughts, beliefs, emotions, habits, and lifestyle, as well as outside influences, all play a role in how you feel on a daily basis, how many daily hassles you have, and if you have muscle tension. Your boss can literally give you a headache, and so can a bad relationship with a loved one or neighbor. It is important to look at all of the contributors to migraine and make adjustments where needed.

Intuition is a valuable gift that needs to be nurtured and trusted to be understood. Your body's intuition can tell you in detail what medical tests cannot, if you are able to hear it.

Understand that there could be one, two, or several issues causing your migraines. No matter which of the healing protocols you need, you also need to include these first three steps—make a commitment to being well—in order to heal and live without head pain.

Make a Commitment to Being Well

There are three important steps to getting well:

1. Believe you will get well.

2. Commit to healing from migraines.

3. Do what it takes to become well.

Step One: Believe

You can control how much oxygen goes to your brain, and you can greatly influence your nervous system and heal it. You can successfully treat your migraines now and, over time, prevent migraines altogether.

For many people, it will take a strong, committed effort and several months or up to a couple of years to be well again. How fast you heal depends on you and the reasons you are having migraines. Healing the liver, blood vessels, neck, or jaw can take time.

I wrote this book to spread the word that you can heal yourself of migraines. You have not only the responsibility, you have the power. Only you can hear your body's messages and make the decisions about your lifestyle and diet that can heal you. It was true for me and for many others I have personally shared my experiences with. It is true for you.

Step Two: Commit

To get well, you need to commit to a new routine and be willing to make good lifestyle choices, which are all outlined in this section. In the process, you may need to change your language to yourself and others.

Making the decision that you are going to become migraine-free is a powerful first step. Decisions are empowering and so is commitment. Say something like this to yourself: "I have decided I am going to live completely free of migraines and I commit to the lifestyle that will allow me to live a strong, vibrant life without pain and limitation." I encourage you to make this commitment now. Write it down and stick to it until your body is healed.

How we express ourselves makes a huge difference. When I had migraines all the time and I was asked how I felt, I would often focus my reply on how the pain in my neck and head felt and how my energy level was. Once I started to get well and knew that it was up to me to be well, I began to talk as if I was already pain-free. I said, "I am doing better all of the time." "I feel great today." "I don't have migraines anymore." I said that before it was true—because I knew the power of words and that our words influence our health, mood, body, and reality. I used the words I wanted to be able to say, in truth.

The words supported my improving health, and my pain diminished. Commit to being well and then commit to it daily with your words and actions. Don't mention migraines because it gives power to the pain instead of to your health. Part of committing to being well is thinking thoughts about being well and speaking as if you are getting well. Your words are powerful and your body will respond to them.

Step Three: Take Action

Once you believe you can heal and you commit to getting well, you will need to take some steps to become healthy and pain-free. Living free of migraines has to do with energy flowing in all areas of the body, without resistance. Stress and poor health slow down the flow. Negative thinking and pressure slow down the flow.

Don't worry about memorizing the information below. It is there for your awareness. You only need to pay attention to the actions to take. For those who want to see the full picture, below are the areas where your flow will increase, and some of the related systems and concepts:

- Oxygen flow (breath)
  - In parasympathetic state with relaxed muscles
- Nerve flow
  - Facia, hydration, spinal alignment, cerebrospinal fluid flow
- Blood flow
  - Liver health and blood vessel health
- Blood vessel health
  - Lymph and blood vessel health
- Liver health
  - Reduced toxicity and healthier blood vessels
- Thought and love flow
  - Emotional and mental awareness
- Minerals
  - Diet and liver health
- Hydration
  - Diet, hydration, liver health, and fascia

The mind, body, and all the systems of the mind and body work together to make you whole.

HOW TO USE THE HEALING PROTOCOLS

This section is intended to be read after you have read the corresponding chapter(s) explaining the physical issue(s) your Migraine Test results indicate.

The three healing protocols are a summary of actions to take based on the test results you had from the beginning of the book. Follow the healing protocol that corresponds with the reason(s) you are having migraines. There are three separate protocols instead of five, because three of the five causes are related. Protocol 1 works for three of the causes of migraines.

If you have a score of 80 or more for L, M, or B, follow the healing guidelines for Protocol 1: liver, minerals, and blood vessels.

If you have a score of 80 or more for H, follow the healing guidelines for Protocol 2: head and neck.

If you have a score of 80 or more for S, follow the healing guidelines for Protocol 3: stress/tension.

Every person is unique in how you will heal and how quickly. My story is one example, but you will heal according to your body, your commitment to getting well, and your current state of health. Migraines are a disease in the body and healing can take time. Be loving and gentle on yourself as you go through this process and know that it is up to you. Also know that you *can* get well, completely.

Your body is telling you, through migraine headaches, that your body has an issue. This is one of the most important lessons I had to learn, and understanding that made it clear to me that taking painkillers was not the solution. I had to fix the problem, not continue to cover it up.

Migraines are the red flag—the indicator
that your body is out of balance.

You will still have migraines after you begin the protocol, but you should notice the level of pain decreasing within two weeks of beginning. Yes, there will be days where you want to reach for the pill that will temporarily give you relief, but that same pill will slow down your healing.

There will be days when you still hate life due to the pain, but be patient. The protocol will help you to deal with pain, reduce the severity of the pain, and heal the nervous system so those pain-filled days will be behind you.

A Note From Diana: What My Healing Journey Looked Like

I had every cause of migraines that is listed in this book. I completed all of these protocols in order to heal completely from migraines. The healing happened with each step I took.

The first step for me was the soft tissue adjustments to my upper cervical vertebrae by a physical therapist, along with neck-strengthening exercises. This immediately helped me travel to altitude without getting a migraine.

The second step was stopping all migraine medication. This was definitely the most difficult step for me. I was taking Sumatriptan 18 times per month and had migraines 25 days per month.

No medication meant near-constant pain for me. But within a week of discontinuing the medication, I had fewer migraines. The month after I stopped taking Sumatriptan, I had 12 days of migraine pain instead of 25 days. The month after that, I had nine days, and the pain was less severe. At that time, I began to watch my consumption of saturated fats, which were contributing to the problem by thickening my blood. I also started to heal my blood vessels with herbs for the vascular system.

The pain and frequency diminished month after month. I continued to get better until I had three to six days of migraine pain per month. Then I hit a plateau.

I didn't learn about relaxing the nervous system through breathing techniques, thoughts, and emotions until later. Once I added the low stress/happy mood component and the perspective of love, I was able to eliminate the migraines altogether. I have learned that some people could start with that aspect and the rest would heal on its own—and that's where part of my Stop, Drop, Roll, and Smile method came from.

Healing my liver took the longest, about two years. From the day I stopped taking Sumatriptan until I no longer had migraines was two and a half years. But I got better every day.

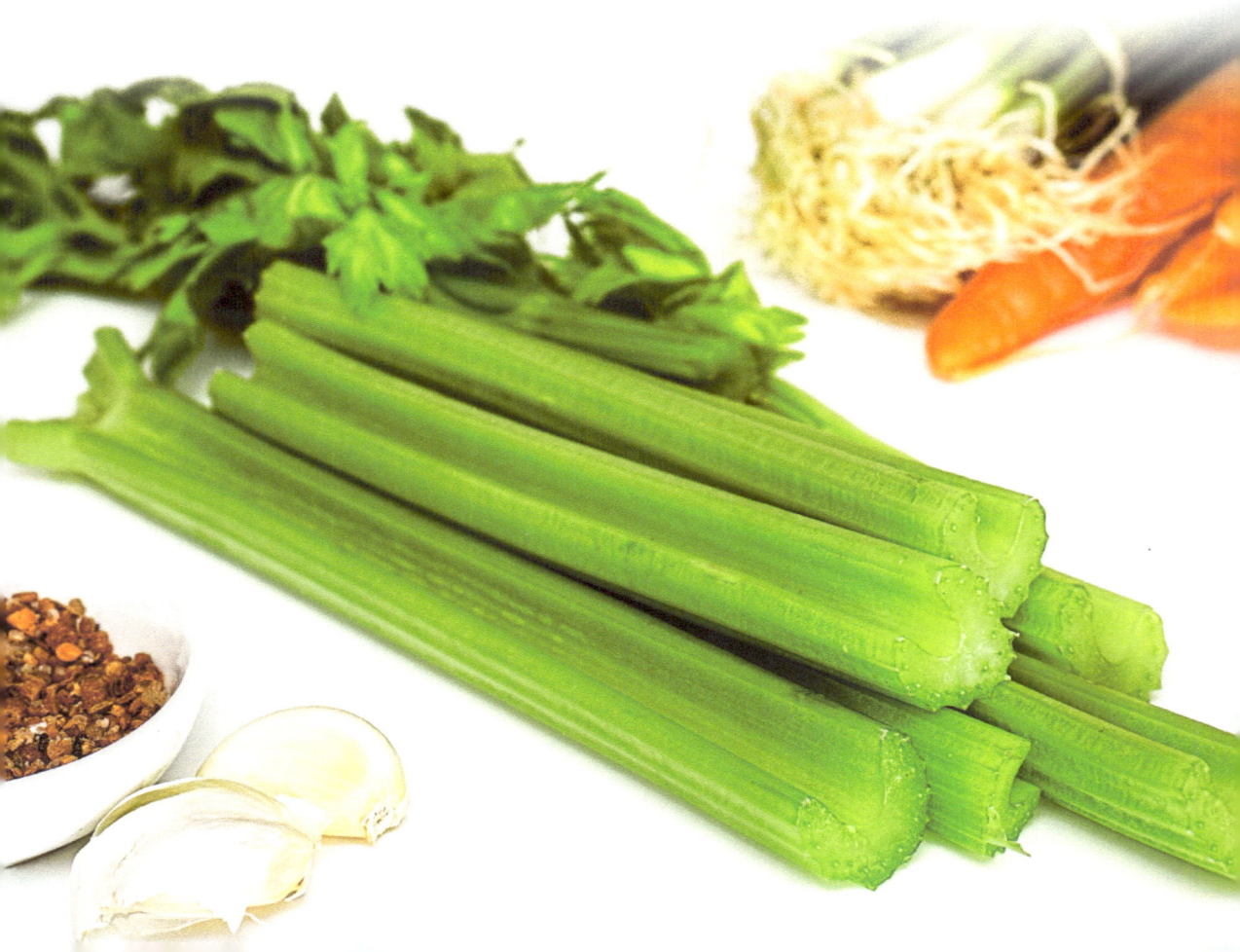

PROTOCOL 1

Liver, Minerals, and Blood Vessels

This protocol works to heal three of the five main causes of low-flow migraines. A toxic or overtaxed liver cannot provide adequate oxygen in the blood. It also affects the availability of minerals, hydration, and glucose, and influences hormone levels, digestion, and more.

A toxic, stagnant, or weak liver does not damage the blood vessels, but healing the blood vessels requires basically the same protocol as healing the liver because blood vessels are damaged by pharmaceutical drugs and/or poor health.

A lack of available minerals may be caused by improper diet or a liver issue; the liver stores and delivers minerals to the blood, which carries the minerals to the parts of the body.

If you score 80 or more for L, M, or B, this protocol can help you become migraine-free.

As you heal your liver, gradually your migraines will decrease in frequency, intensity, and duration. If you notice fewer migraines, or less intense and shorter migraines, you can celebrate because your liver is recovering. This can take years, as it did for me, depending on how much damage or stagnation your liver has and how well you follow a protocol that will aid your liver's health. It is worth every effort you make. Even a small improvement in the health of your liver will improve the quality of your life.

Some of the steps that follow require the help of an alternative medicine practitioner. Find a reputable Chinese medical practitioner, naturopath, osteopath, or other functional medical practitioner through personal referral, if at all possible. This can speed up your healing.

Understand that a healthy person (who does not suffer from migraines) does not have to go to these lengths in terms of eliminating toxins, taking supplements, and limiting food triggers. The low flow condition makes your body hypersensitive to blood or oxygen fluctuations and these steps will help reduce the inflammation and allow your systems to heal.

You may find it helpful to keep a daily journal to record headache pain and also the foods you eat, especially if you already know you have food triggers. The journal will help you track the frequency of your pain and also pinpoint any new headache triggers (foods, weather, specific events) or anything that seems to help, such as exercise, particular supplements, massage, etc.

Step 1: Eliminate Toxins

Eliminate your exposure to toxins, mold, poisons, and chemicals. Check your home and work environments for exposure to any toxin that the body must flush out regularly. These include cleaning chemicals, pesticides and herbicides, smoke from cigarettes, oil-based paints and varnishes, and many health and beauty products such as nail polish and hair dyes.

While your liver is struggling to keep up, it needs time to heal with a reprieve from the chemicals that harm the body. Your liver's job is to remove these problematic substances from your blood so they don't harm your cells. When it is overtaxed, the liver can't get all the work done. If you can stay away from as many chemicals as possible, your liver can rest and renew. Here are some of the things that will help, and there are many more to consider that are not on this list.

- Purchase natural cleaning products or have someone else handle the cleaning.
- Have someone else handle pesticides or consider not using them in and around your home.

- Do not paint your nails until your liver works well.

- Stay away from certain hair products like dyes and some hair sprays. Aveda hair products are made with natural essential oils and I have used them without issue.

- Assist your liver by eating foods that are natural, such as fruits and veggies and less-processed foods. Your liver works hard to take chemicals out of junk food so the cells can have only nourishment.

- Have your home checked for mold, radon, and other toxic chemicals.

- Avoid using products like paint, stain, and varnish.

You cannot heal the liver without giving it a reprieve from toxins, both physical and emotional. Negative emotions can cause the body to release stress hormones. Process, heal, and release old emotions of anger and resentment, which are held in the liver. This is an Eastern medicine practice and it was an important part of my own healing process, although it was difficult for me to accept it at first.

The emotional toxins take more effort to overcome, but if you have habitual negative emotions, this is an important step for you to truly heal all sources of your migraine pain. Work to avoid negative thinking, anger, and other toxic emotions.

Toxins of many types add to the load your liver must process. Your health will begin to improve once you stop adding fuel to the fire of a toxic liver.

Step 2: Eliminate Pharmaceutical Medications and Anti-Inflammatory Drugs

Stop taking all pain medications, whether prescription or OTC, and any other pharmaceutical drug you can be without. Avoid all anti-inflammatory drugs, triptans, antihistamines, and decongestants.

With the help of your doctor, avoid any drug that expands or contracts your blood vessels. Even if you must stay on some medications, lightening the load of prescriptions and eliminating all alcohol and OTC drugs will start moving your liver health in the right direction. Long-term use of these drugs causes damage to the vascular muscle walls, especially common NSAIDs (such as ibuprofen) and opiate painkillers.

There are many pain management systems to help you deal with migraine pain during your healing. Start with the *Stop, Drop, Roll, and Smile* pain management protocol included in this book.

Note: Some patients will need to continue use of some medications for high blood pressure or heart issues. Consult your doctor before stopping use of prescription drugs.

Step 3: Find a Mild Liver Cleanse

Consult a qualified traditional Chinese medicine doctor who can help you treat your liver or do a mild, gentle liver cleanse that is tailored to your health condition. Some herbal cleanses are valuable, however which herbs are helpful depends on your level of health and the cause and type of your liver stagnation. Be very careful with what you read and practice regarding liver cleansing.

Do not drink olive oil, or any oil, as part of a liver cleanse. Both Western and Eastern medicine recommend that you don't practice severe and stressful cleansing of the liver. I enjoyed the easy 28-day liver cleanse diet described in *Liver Rescue* by Anthony William.

Step 4: Liquid Minerals and Herbal Supplements for Blood Vessels

Until the liver is well, eat a healthy diet. Take liquid minerals and eat celery. Celery is very high in many minerals. I recommend getting a high-quality brand of mineral supplement from a reputable health food store and notice if it helps you. You may need to try a few brands to find one that reduces headache pain.

I found great success with the brand NOW Colloidal Minerals. It consists of a large number of the body's trace and major minerals. I felt the difference when I took this, as it improved my hydration and made my head feel less "hot" and less painful. When I used to get restless legs at night, I sometimes took these minerals and the issue stopped within two minutes.

Be sure to drink plenty of water when taking liquid minerals—and in general. Hydration is key to all protocols for improving your health and eliminating migraines.

In addition to liver health, for blood vessel healing, stopping all prescription and OTC medications is the first crucial step. The second is to actively support the healing process. Hawthorn berry and other herbs including feverfew and ginkgo biloba have been prescribed in their unaltered plant form for over 3,000 years in Eastern medicine to heal the heart and blood vessels. Your Chinese medicine practitioner may also have an herbal mixture for this purpose. Although Western medicine does not recognize these herbs as effective, Eastern medicine does, as do alternative medicine approaches.

Consult your medical doctor and also educate yourself before taking any herbs, as they may interfere with other medication you might be taking.

Step 5: Limit Food Triggers and Focus on Blood-Thinning, Nutrient-Dense Foods

Be conscious of how much saturated fat, blood-thickening foods, and toxins (in the form of processed foods) you eat every day. Especially if you have food triggers for your migraines, I recommend not more than one meal with butter, other animal fat, or nut butter per day. Also avoid all alcohol, including wine and beer, as they thicken the blood and reduce hydration. As you heal, you can gradually add these things back in.

See the Food List in the Appendix for foods to eat more of and foods to avoid. Foods to eat more of are blood-thinning foods and those with the nutrients you need—glucose and minerals.

If you have any food addictions or you need a cleanse, I recommend the cleanse described in Anthony William's book *Liver Rescue*. It is a 28-day cleanse that consists of all the fruits and veggies you can eat. I never felt hungry because I could eat all of the fruits and vegetables I wanted. I had good energy the whole time and I felt more energized afterward. Although changing the diet is not easy or fun, it will quickly reduce migraines and the tradeoff is well worth the gain in vitality.

Eat a lot of fruit and anti-inflammatory foods. These help you to stay hydrated and feed your brain natural glucose combined with minerals.

Chinese medicine recognizes a few different causes of a stagnant or weak liver. A different diet is often recommended, depending on which cause of liver dysfunction you have. Ask your Chinese doctor what your cause of liver weakness is and follow their diet and lifestyle recommendations.

Step 6: Self-Care

While you heal your liver, you need to increase hydration and blood flow throughout your body. Try the following and see what helps you.

- *Make quality hydration your new habit.* This includes spring water, unpolluted water, coconut water, freshly squeezed orange or other juices, and watermelon. You may be somewhat dehydrated on a daily basis without realizing it, especially if you drink caffeinated beverages, like coffee and tea, or alcohol, such as wine or beer. Be sure to drink at least one glass of water for every cup of coffee or tea, and consider cutting back on caffeinated beverages. Avoid *all* alcohol.

- Eat a diet high in vegetables, fruits, antioxidants, ginger, turmeric, and omega-3 fats. Fruit is not the same as processed sugar and should not be categorized with sugar. See the Understanding Oxygen, Minerals, and Glucose section below.

- Gentle exercise, sunshine, stretching, and avoiding prolonged sitting are all habits you should develop. This includes walking and bouncing to stimulate flow. See the Understanding Lymph Flow section below.

- Gentle massage helps the lymph. Stronger massage can stimulate blood flow. See the Understanding Lymph Flow section below.

- Spend time each day resting the nervous system from external stimulation. During this time, avoid electronic devices, talking with others, and what is happening outside of yourself. Go within to your internal world and just be—listening to your breathing. This is where healing happens. Read the section in **Protocol 3** on Stress and Tension. This will help you regardless of the underlying causes of your migraines.

Understanding Lymph Flow

Helping the lymph to flow properly helps blood flow and supports the liver. Things that specifically influence lymph flow are listed here:

- Movement, walking, yoga, twisting and stretching the spine, exercise, getting your heart rate up, and bouncing on a rebounder or large trampoline.

- Sweating during any activity, including sitting in an infrared sauna.

- Light-touch massage, flowing toward the center of the body, done by yourself or others, or frequent massage.

- Topical treatments using essential oils on the skin to promote blood circulation.

  · Arnica cream helps relax and heal muscles.

  · Peppermint in the bathtub promotes deeper breathing and blood flow.

  · Menthol promotes pain relief, breathing, and blood flow.

  · Lavender calms the nervous system.

  · Essential oils can be purchased at the local health food store and online. Always buy high quality brands. White Flower Oil is a combination of essential oils and menthol, which I have had great success with. This product is available on Amazon and at many health food stores.

  · Castor oil is helpful when used topically on sore muscles. It has properties that aren't fully understood, but it is excellent for supporting the lymph system. Castor oil is also used over the liver as a compact to support liver health and support liver function. I recommend it *for topical use only*. It can be purchased online or at a health food store.

Understanding Oxygen, Minerals, and Glucose

You may think "hydration" means drinking enough water. However, without the proper balance of minerals in your cells, water cannot enter. Minerals allow the fluid to enter as well as exit your cells, and both processes—entering and exiting—are critical for proper hydration. Your liver provides minerals to your bloodstream and then to the cells and if it is not functioning properly, you can be dehydrated in spite of drinking plenty of water.

The liver stores minerals and supplies them to the blood, so the long-term fix for hydration is healing the liver from toxins and eating a healthy diet. Until your liver is functioning as it should, you can increase your hydration through *super hydration*—by consuming oranges, watermelon, and coconut water as well as high-quality mineral supplements, and drinking large amounts of quality mineral water.

Also avoid foods that dehydrate the body: crackers, bread, dry foods, foods high in saturated fats, and any food that will take water from your cells in order to digest it. When you choose what you eat, remember the analogy of washing food down a drain. How much water would it take to wash coconut water down a drain? None. How much water would it take to wash coconut oil down a drain? A lot. Ingest a lot of coconut water or fruit, not coconut oil or butter.

Note on Supplements

For a full list of the few supplements and all the foods I recommend, refer to the Food List in the Appendix. I do not advocate taking a lot of supplements. Getting nutrients from food helps you regulate the amounts. When you are low on something and while you are healing, you can use supplements to provide the needed resources until your body is back in balance.

In Conclusion: The Liver, Minerals, and Blood Vessels

Having a healthy liver is critical to having a pain-free life. If you do nothing else to heal yourself from migraines, heal the liver. Most likely, it is the most important step for you to live a pain-free life.

PROTOCOL 2

Head and Neck

Spinal health, alignment, and strength is vital to living free of pain. Head, neck, and spinal injuries can impinge on nerves through inflammation or narrowed pathways and affect the flow of blood, lymph, and cerebrospinal fluid to your head. This reduced flow of resources is a critical part of the low flow condition that can cause migraine headaches.

If you scored 80 or higher in the H column of the Migraine Test, this protocol can help you become migraine-free.

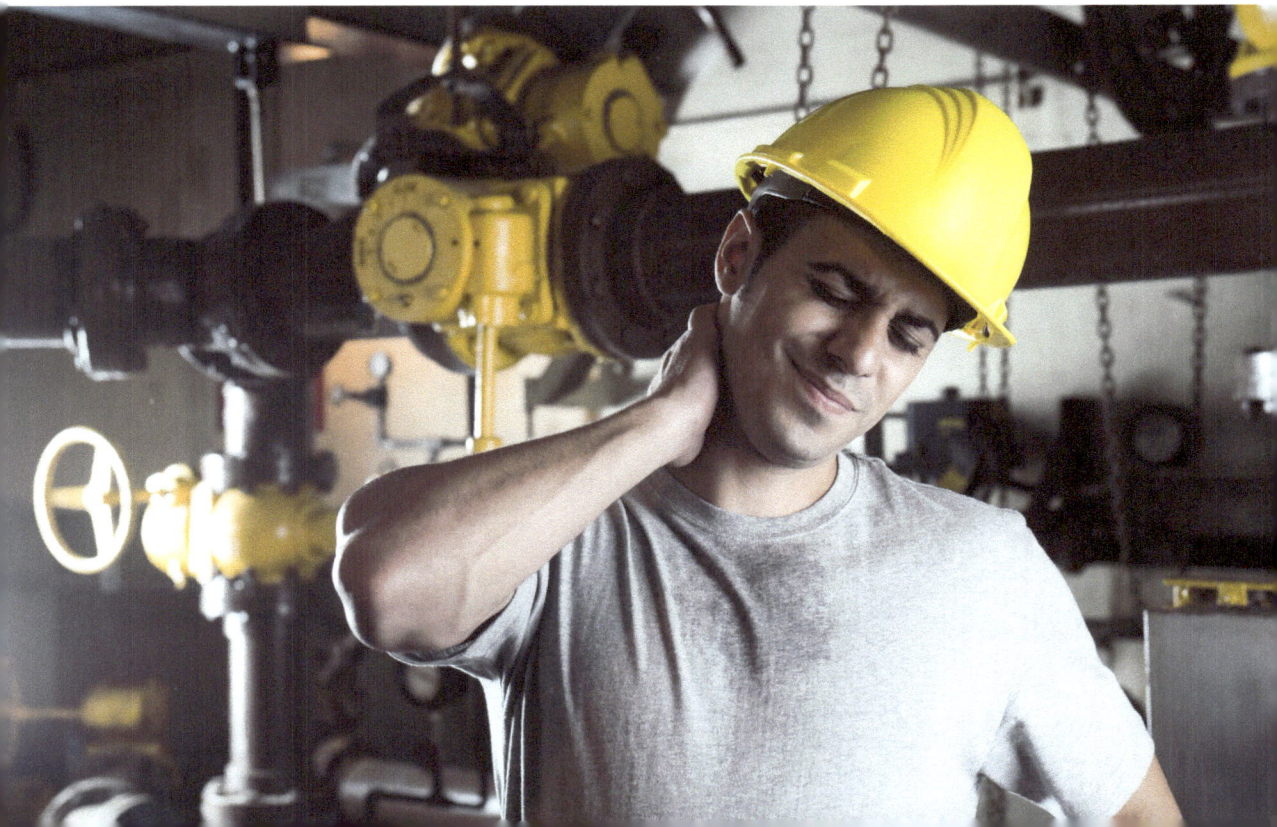

Alignment of the Spine Is Alignment With the Self and the Spirit

Posture is as powerful as positive thinking. Good spinal alignment permits proper nerve energy flow, which allows the entire nervous system, including the brain, to work better. How you sit, walk, and stand can determine whether you have headaches. I invite you to look at all areas of your life that affect the nervous system, spinal alignment, and muscle tension.

Step 1: Align and Heal Your Neck and Spine

If you have had head or neck injuries or surgeries, you may need the help of a specialist who can do soft tissue manipulation. This will help to realign your neck and relieve impingement on nerves and flow. Look for one of these professionals:

- Osteopath
- Chiropractor
- Doctor of Physical Therapy (DPT)
- Physical therapist with additional training: Orthopedic Certified Specialist (OCS)
- Physical therapist with this specialty: Fellow of Applied Functional Science (FAFS), Gray Institute

This healthcare provider can also help you with identifying where you have weakness and providing exercises to strengthen those muscles.

The Process of Neck Healing

Neck healing happens in three stages. First, get rid of inflammation. Second, align and stabilize. Third, build strength to maintain stability.

Eliminate Inflammation in the Neck

To eliminate inflammation, the neck must be properly aligned. So your first step is to find a physical therapist who can help you with soft tissue adjustment for immediate relief. A diet low in inflammatory foods and a low stress lifestyle will help reduce the inflammation in your spine.

Align and Stabilize the Neck

The physical therapist/osteopath who helps you with alignment can prescribe exercises that will help your neck become stronger and more stable and teach you ways to keep it in alignment. Healthy movements and regular relaxation are an important part of staying in alignment.

Address all impingements on blood and lymph flow: See your osteo/physical therapist twice per month or as needed, to make small adjustments to your spine for about three to six months, until your cervical vertebrae have stabilized and are staying in place for longer periods of time.

Do the neck, trapezius muscle, and any mid-back exercises prescribed by your physical therapist for a few days per week. These will help to stabilize your neck and strengthen your upper back. Stretch your spine daily. These exercises may need to become lifelong habits to maintain the health of your neck and spine.

After the inflammation in your neck has improved, you can do many things to keep your spine healthy:

1. Relaxation, stress management/deep breathing. Relax neck muscles to assist in blood flow. Deep relaxation is highly valuable and takes practice. It is one of the most valuable things you can learn.

2. Stretching, moving, dancing, and exercising will all help blood to circulate in the back and neck.

3. Be aware of your posture, relax your shoulders and jaw, align your spine. Notice if your shoulders rise when you reach away from your body. If they do, your neck muscles could be weak and your body is tightening the shoulders to compensate. Discuss this with your physical therapist/osteopath. Experiment with different bed pillows to allow for proper neck support.

4. Notice if you have difficulty breathing slowly and deeply. It could be related to spinal misalignment. Deep relaxation can often improve alignment without needing any adjustment by a chiropractor or therapist, but you must reach a state of deeply

relaxing the neck muscles. Tight muscles can pull your spine and neck out of alignment.

5. Rest and relax the jaw if you have tight or painful jaw muscles. Eat soft food, avoid gum chewing, choose times to stop talking, and practice leaving the jaw open and relaxed. Perform jaw exercises to stretch and relax the jaw muscles. You will have to train your jaw to stay relaxed during the day. *If you have a tight jaw, it is contributing to your migraines!*

6. Use an ergonomic setup at the computer with good posture, taking care to not stretch the upper back muscles and keeping conscious to engage the correct muscles.

7. If you get tight, painful points on your back, do *trigger point release* or massage. For trigger point release, lie on the floor on your back. Place one or more tennis balls under your back, on the painful point. Gently and slowly roll the tennis ball(s) across your back while lying on them to force the trigger point to relax. Using the tennis ball to press hard on the muscle that is too tight cuts off some circulation temporarily. Then when you release the pressure, it floods the area with blood, allowing the muscle to relax a little. This can end a cycle of continuous contraction that causes the muscle to get so tight.

8. Do Qigong breathing exercises and hold the relaxation wrist points. These two practices work rapidly, relieving tension and pain in 10 minutes very effectively.

Build Strength in the Neck

Again, work with your physical therapist/osteopath to strengthen your neck and back muscles for long-term neck and spinal health.

Step 2: Deep Breathing

Deep breathing is especially important if you have pinched nerves or impingement in your neck or spine. You need to learn how to do it properly and make this your habitual breathing mode. Deep breathing is one of the most effective ways to prevent the nervous system from going into flight-or-flight mode, which can lead to a migraine. Also, being aware of your breathing can help you identify when your neck or spine is out of alignment.

How to practice deep breathing is described near the beginning of Section Two. Also visit my website at RealMigraineSolutions.com or go to YouTube for my videos on how to perform deep breathing.

Step 3: Relax Your Muscles

Tight muscles can pull your neck or spine out of alignment. Daily stresses or unusual stresses can cause you to tighten your muscles. Especially if you have neck or spine issues, you need to know how to relax your muscles.

Jaw Tightness

Jaw tightness due to TMJ issues, tension, or habitual gritting or grinding of the teeth can cause tight muscles in the jaw and across the back of the head.

In order to relax, you need to be *present* with your body. Here is a practice to try: Spend time becoming aware of what is happening to your body when neck pain and head pain begin. This tension can be caused by pressure to hurry or perform, or by talking, chewing, etc., and then your neck can be pulled out of place by tight muscles. On some occasions, maybe your neck gets out of alignment first and then muscles tighten up to compensate for the misalignment and your jaw muscles tighten also. Other times the tension can begin in the low back or buttocks and creep up the spine, all the way to the jaw, especially when you're dehydrated and your fascia gets tight.

Learn to consciously relax your muscles. Start with the jaw and work your way down to your feet. Feel the muscles as each area releases. The tension may let go in a specific order and the low back or buttocks may be the last muscles to release the tension. Sometimes the tension begins at the bottom of the spine and moves to the top of the head. Then when the release happens, the muscles release in reverse, from the top of the head to the buttocks.

Address Your Trigger Points

Having a few trigger points here and there is usually just an annoyance. Having many can lead to a migraine. See the links below on how to address trigger points, if you have them.

https://www.painscience.com/tutorials/trigger-points.php

https://www.painscience.com/articles/self-massage.php

Creating Strong Blood Flow to the Head

The best remedy to improve neck and back alignment is to do exercises prescribed by a physical therapist to strengthen the muscles and keep them working properly. As the alignment improves and muscles strengthen, muscle tension will subside. As the muscles relax, blood and oxygen flow to the head will increase.

Work to keep your spine aligned. Improving your posture starts with strengthening the gluteus maximus muscles through butt exercises, lengthening the hip flexors with stretches, and improving your neck posture with exercises to prevent forward neck syndrome.

Work in an ergonomically neutral position as much as possible, including a standing desk, and take frequent stretching/moving exercise breaks.

Reducing demands and pressure in your schedule must be a part of your health routine. Tension and anxiety also contribute to neck and back misalignment by tightening the neck muscles and pulling the spine out of alignment.

Step 4: Self-Care

For some people, the shingles or Epstein-Bar virus can impact nerves that increase neck and head pain. If you believe viruses may play a role in your neck pain and/or your migraines, consult with your Chinese medicine practitioner or other herbal expert to discover if a lobelia tincture or other treatment may help to eliminate the viruses from your body.

For severe neck pain, get in the tub, lather your neck with castor oil, and sit there as long as you can. It helps take away the pain and promotes circulation of the lymph and blood.

Support your health with an anti-inflammatory diet (not to be confused with OTC anti-inflammatory drugs. Ask your nutritional expert for recommendations for healing foods to help you improve your health).

Understanding Chiropractors and Physical Therapists

On occasion, we can benefit from being adjusted by a chiropractor or therapist. However, relying on only a chiropractor for adjustments is not enough. It is possible that over a long period of time, chiropractic adjustments to C1 and C2 can further strain and weaken the ligaments that hold the vertebrae in proper alignment.

A more long-term solution toward neck and spinal health is to find a qualified physical therapist or osteopath. These healthcare professionals specialize in the muscles and tendons that support your body.

A physical therapist can evaluate you and show you the exercises that are right for you. Almost every person can benefit from aligning neck exercises because forward neck syndrome is so prevalent today, not only in injured people but also for those who work at a computer or desk every day or spend time looking at their cell phones.

If finances are an issue and prevent you from seeing a specialist, you can try neck strengthening exercises, good spinal movement, and deep relaxation as I describe, and you may get the results you want. If you want to try it on your own first, I also recommend trying Qigong for a few weeks and seeing how you feel.

Diana's Story

A fellow hiker who was hiking with me and noticed I couldn't take the altitude change in the Santa Barbara hills just happened to be a physical/osteo therapist. He said he could help. I took a chance and made an appointment. With each visit and the gentle soft-tissue adjustments and neck manipulation he did, my daily migraines were reduced so drastically that people noticed how much better I looked and felt. I also did all of the recommended neck, hip, and back exercises to strengthen my neck and properly align my spine. The exercises trained me to use my muscles correctly, which created stability in my spine. The exercises also increased my spinal fluid movement, which added nourishment to the nerves in my neck and head.

On many occasions, I noticed that I was not able to consistently change my breathing into slow, deep belly breaths, no matter how hard I tried. I realized that my neck was out of alignment and the pinched nerve was triggering the autonomic nervous system to respond in a fight-or-flight manner. Even when I tried to override the system consciously with a longer exhale, it didn't usually work. I eventually found methods for re-aligning my neck and getting the muscles to relax, and once I did that, I was able to change my breathing to deep belly breathing.

Neck Realignment Methods

If you suspect you have a neck alignment issue that prevents you from truly relaxing with deep belly breathing, here are some of the methods I learned to prevent the oncoming headache:

1. Stop working on the computer. Lie down and meditate, and relax all neck and jaw muscles. Allow the mouth to salivate. Then hang your head upside down, free from using any muscles, and wiggle it with your hand to align it. Do this without engaging neck muscles.

2. Rest your neck muscles by taking the weight of the head off of the neck muscles. Do this by lying on your back on your bed or on the floor. Then your neck muscles are not working and you can get them to relax. Breathe slowly and deeply and let go of all stress and muscle tension.

3. Make sure the jaw muscles are relaxed as well, and smile a little. Think of things you are grateful for to encourage serotonin flow, which increases blood flow to the nervous system as well.

4. Take liquid minerals, spray on liquid magnesium oil, or take a mineral bath and massage your neck muscles. Or use White Flower Oil (see Supplements and Sources in the Appendix).

5. Do Qigong breathing exercises and hold the relaxation wrist points. These two things work rapidly, relieving tension and pain in 10 minutes, very effectively.

In Conclusion: Head and Neck

Working on your posture, strengthening neck and back muscles, and being kind to your spine will all help ensure that you won't have pinched nerves and blood vessels. Long-term spinal health comes from training the neck muscles to do the work through specific exercises and improving posture. This is far more empowering than simply getting aligned by manipulation. Spinal health is one of the very best things you can do for yourself.

You may also need to teach your body a "new normal" to prevent the autonomic fight-or-flight stress response if you have chronic neck issues. Do this through deep breathing and meditation or other focused relaxation techniques.

NOTE: A less common cause of migraine happens from spinal fluid slowly leaking from the spinal column at the junctures where nerves exit the spine. Highly specialized medical treatment can assist people with this issue, which is not addressed here. Symptoms often include frequent, ongoing migraines. This is worth noting for those who do not find relief from the material in this protocol. Anytime spinal fluid is low, cortisol is released, which triggers fight or flight.

All migraines
happen when you
are in fight-or-flight
mode.

PROTOCOL 3

Stress and Tension

You will never have a headache when your nervous system is in a state of rest and digest, also called the parasympathetic state. I'll say this another way: the surest way to prevent or eliminate a headache is to be in a parasympathetic state and avoid fight or flight, the sympathetic state. Stress can cause your body to remain in fight-or-flight mode as your "normal" daily mode. This has long-term health consequences and can be the cause of your migraines. This protocol focuses on methods you can use the change your body's normal stress response and find a new normal.

If you scored 80 or higher in the S column of the Migraine Test, this protocol can help you become migraine-free.

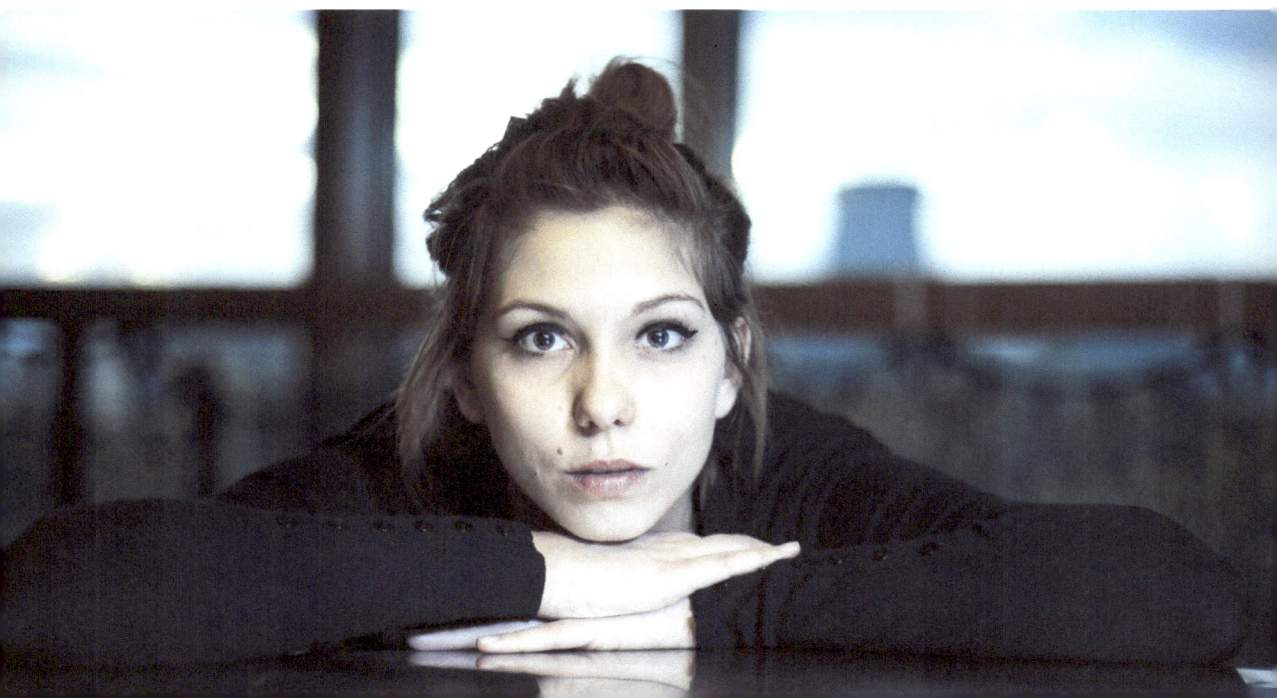

Step 1: Learn to Relax

If stress is one of the causes for your migraines, reducing worry and demands is critical to good health and less head pain. Learning how to deliberately relax yourself both physically and mentally, telling your body *there is no emergency*, is key to preventing and relieving headaches. You are much less likely to have a migraine headache if you are getting enough downtime, breathing properly, exercising regularly, and are not under pressure at work—financially or emotionally. If you have ongoing pressure in your work or life that you can't resolve, then your task becomes finding a way to recognize what you can't control and escape the stress those circumstances cause. You may need professional help or conversations with a mentor or confidant to achieve reframing your circumstances in a positive way.

Part of learning to relax is becoming aware of your body and noticing if you are holding tension in your muscles. Throughout the day, it is a good practice to notice your jaw, neck, back, and shoulder muscles. Notice your breathing and become aware of how your thoughts impact your body functions. Then practice relaxing muscles with intention and deep breathing. Focus on an area and intentionally relax it as you feel the muscle let go, little by little, until the tension is gone.

The human body is designed to take periods of rest, and that reprieve will be truly effective if your mind and your muscles are relaxed. Practice feelings of satisfaction and gratitude so your body releases serotonin, which relaxes the nervous system and muscles, allowing for blood to flow to the brain. When you are practicing relaxation and being present, find those muscles in your body that seem tense or painful and work on ways to relax them. This may require massage or targeted stretching exercises you do at home or work. If you need assistance learning how, you can enlist the help of a professional, until you can do it yourself.

See **Protocol 2,** Step 3 for more information. Visit RealMigraineSolutions.com and my YouTube channel for videos on relaxation and deep breathing.

Step 2: Deep Breathing

If you are thinking the deep breathing keeps coming up, you are correct. It can help with any form of migraine. Revisit the Deep Breathing exercises at the beginning of Section Two for the details on how to do this.

When you are in a parasympathetic state, your breathing is slow and relaxed. Your mind is *present* with what is happening in the moment, and you are not thinking much about the future or the past—you are here, now. In this state, you feel calm and grateful, without fear of financial issues, relationship problems, or health concerns. Achieving this state is worth the effort because it helps not only your mental state but your entire physical state as well.

If you do have ongoing concerns about something, you must deliberately let them go for a while, to move the nervous system into a state where it can relax and help you let your guard down. A sign that you are relaxed is when saliva accumulates in your mouth. This is proven to calm the nervous system and is a sign to the body that all is well. If your mouth is very dry—and not dry from medications or dehydration—then you likely have tension. When you are relaxed enough to salivate, you will naturally have less pain.

Step 3: Make Correct Breathing a Habit

If you are getting frequent migraines, there is a 90 percent chance you are not breathing deeply and slowly, using your diaphragm, as your normal way to breathe. This deep breathing is what I mean by correct breathing. When you breathe correctly, you send the right signals to your nervous system that all is well, you are calm, and the body can focus on delivering blood to your brain.

> Breathing correctly is key to living migraine-free.

You may still need to heal your liver, blood vessels, and blood if you have multiple causes of your migraines, but in the meantime, proper breathing will aid your body in good oxygen delivery and keep your nervous system out of fight-or-flight mode. This is a first step toward preventing migraines and it aids greatly in the healing process.

Sometimes you may struggle to breathe properly, even when you deliberately try. That is because if the body feels threatened from a pinched nerve, low glucose, low CSF, or cold temperatures, it can choose to stay in a sympathetic state to protect the body. In that state, breathing is automatically shallow, even when you consciously try to breathe deeply and slowly. I discussed this phenomenon in **Protocol 2** in my story and under Neck Realignment Methods, and it can happen for any of the reasons that threaten the resource supply to the brain.

To avoid a headache, you will need to continue to try to override the system by relaxing the jaw and taking slow, deep breaths, getting back to a parasympathetic state of feeling relaxed and safe. This can take minutes or it can take hours.

Step 4: Examine Your Attitudes

I have explained to several migraine sufferers that they must stop, drop, roll, and smile the minute they feel a migraine coming on. Every one of them said, "I don't have time to stop and deal with a migraine. I have too much to do, no time to rest, stretch, breathe, or take care of myself." ***This is the attitude that sets the ball in motion to start a migraine in the first place.***

"No time" triggers the fight-or-flight response, which directs less oxygen to the brain. Rushing can trigger muscle tension or push a weak neck out of alignment. If you feel that you don't have time for a break when a migraine starts, think about the downtime you will have from the migraine that is coming. Migraines can last for three days. The hangover from the migraine can last at least a day. If you don't have time to stop, then you also don't have time to allow a migraine to take hold.

A 20-minute break could save you up to three or four days of pain and time away from work and life. Study the four steps in the Stop, Drop, Roll, and Smile method for reducing or eliminating headaches and find a way to make the time for this when you feel a headache coming on.

Ways to Calm the Body and Stimulate the Vagus Nerve

In order to live without head pain that is caused by stress, you must retrain yourself on the art of relaxation. This means communicating through your vagus nerve. The vagus nerve communicates that all is well to the autonomic nervous system—and it also communicates when it is *not* well.

Practicing deep breathing and relaxation can communicate through the vagus nerve that it's okay to relax. After all, a migraine is, in effect, a forced rest. If you rest well naturally, then you won't be forced by your body and brain to take the needed reprieve.

We all relax differently. It took me a long time to learn how to begin the shift from fight or flight into rest and digest. Once you know how it feels to have this level of calm, you will naturally find your own ways to achieve that peace.

The skill of consciously telling your body to relax, of communicating to your autonomic nervous system, is extremely helpful in healing your body and alleviating migraines.

Regardless of the underlying causes, it's that added stress of being in the sympathetic state of emergency (fight or flight) that depletes your brain's resources to the point that a migraine develops. I keep repeating this because it's so important to understand.

Deep breathing is the starting point for all of the exercises below. Learn what kinds of actions and thoughts help you to feel good. Consider the list that follows as a starting point and use what works for you.

1. **Breathe deeply and immerse your tongue in saliva.** Do this by completely relaxing your jaw, lips, checks, face muscles, neck, and eyes. Bathe your tongue in saliva while breathing deeply through your nose. Enjoy the feelings of relaxation in your head, neck, hands, hips, and feet. Do this for three minutes or longer. Don't cheat yourself on the time.

2. **Think about loved ones.** As you breathe, feel love for someone close to you, even a pet. Think of how you feel because you love them so much. Think of ways you want to make them happy

and things you can do for them or things you enjoy doing with them. Do this for at least 10 minutes. This will relax your systems and cause your breathing to naturally relax. It will also increase hormones that promote good circulation. Try the same exercise with another person that you love. It can also help to touch a pet or someone that you love. It is effective if done in a relaxed manner, forgetting all other cares. Feeling love and gratitude for people in your life changes your state and slows down your breathing.

3. **Smile.** Hold a slight smile for as long as you can. The act of smiling releases the hormone serotonin, which positively affects blood flow to the brain and helps calm the entire nervous system. Smiling can reverse a migraine if there are enough resources available, i.e., hydration, minerals, oxygen, and glucose.

4. **Gentle self-massage.** If no one is around to touch you, caress your own skin in a kind, loving way. Caress your face, neck, and arms slowly for several minutes, breathing in deeply as you do this and sighing on the release of your breath. Do this for five minutes. If you are at work, this may be difficult to do. Whenever possible, get out in nature where the earth's energy helps you become more grounded and balanced. Find a quiet place to massage your hands and give yourself soothing touch while you breathe. It is very effective if you do this calmly for several minutes. This gets your awareness into your body and helps you to be grounded. Being grounded is one of the fastest ways to calm the nervous system, which is an electrical system that must be grounded to function optimally. The earth is our natural, giant grounding system, but plants, rocks, and water can be brought inside to help ground us in small ways. Being grounded can be as simple as bringing your awareness to your body and/or nature around you. You can also watch YouTube videos on ways to calm your nervous system. Find a practice that works well for you.

Find a New Normal

You may need to learn a *new normal* state and teach yourself how good it feels to be relaxed. Try having a deeply relaxing massage and then notice how it feels to be so relaxed. Try to memorize this relaxed feeling so you can recall it when you need to unwind. Do activities that calm you the most and notice how that feels.

Rest and digest is also referred to as "grow and renew," or the healing state. Without downtime and relaxation, people age faster, and healing is greatly impaired. Take time to relax and your total health will improve!

However, muscle relaxing medications are *not* the answer. The forced relaxation from muscle relaxants is a façade and does not accomplish what you want. Instead of taking muscle relaxants, see your physical therapist and strengthen all of the muscles in your back. Learn many relaxation techniques and find the ones that work for you.

Improve your posture. Good posture is powerful in keeping the body's energy flow at its best. Sometimes this fundamental necessity to good health is underestimated.

Whether the cause is mental, emotional, or physical stress, you have to learn what it feels like to be completely relaxed and know what works for you to generate that feeling at will. It is worth the effort. You will have some degree of pain in your body until you can find a way to be completely relaxed.

The Power of Meditation

The health benefits of meditation are widely documented. Yet getting motivated to dedicate time to this practice can be a challenge.

Meditation is highly beneficial to the nervous system, giving it a time to rest, recuperate, and recover. No matter what the cause of a migraine, stress always will make it worse. Mediation is the opposite of stress. It is the water to put out the fire.

Start With Being Present

Many people struggle to meditate, finding it challenging to quiet their mind. If you struggle with it, a simpler form of meditation you can try is simply being *present.* Meditation is about focusing on being present. You are present with your breath, a sound, or a body sensation. If focusing on one of those things is too difficult and your mind always wonders, try staying focused on something easy for you. That could be painting, sewing, doing a favorite sport, or cuddling with your partner. If you are present while you are actively engaged in an activity, that is very close to deep mediation and it will offer you many benefits.

Meditation Takes Practice

Once you have practiced staying present, you might be able to move into a meditation practice. It may take one hour to declutter your mind at the start. After many attempts, it may take 30 minutes. Eventually, you can jump into deep meditation in one minute as your body and mind memorize the state and quickly drop into the pattern.

Deep meditation has big advantages, including a feeling of total and absolute bliss. This state is very healing to the entire body. Once in the blissful state, you can focus your awareness on a part of your body and invoke healing to that part of the body. Focus on it for a period of time and notice all of the sensations that come up.

Consciously Avoid Becoming Stressed

Consciously practice accepting daily stresses and pressures as a part of your life so they don't upset you. Getting upset is definitely a contributor to headaches. Consciously decide that those stresses are a normal part of your life instead of a reason for panic or irritation.

Feeling stressed about deadlines and meetings, client expectations, or family can easily trigger all of the bodily functions that contribute to headaches. Be aware of this and force yourself to breathe, relax, allow what is happening to just happen, and don't resist. Think positively and don't let outside circumstances bother you, as much as you possibly can.

Learn positive reframing techniques to handle challenging issues. Positive thinking methods, calming techniques, and reframing your perspective to control stressful thoughts all help to change the patterns that cause mental stress.

Thought patterns of worry, doubt, fear, and low self-esteem can tense the body. If your circulation is compromised from any other causes, such as a taxed liver, then mental stress can quickly turn into a headache.

Seek Brain and Body Coherence

When your mental awareness is fully present with your physical body and current situation, without distracting thoughts, the body and brain go into a matching rhythm we refer to as *coherence,* which is a state that allows for proper flow of blood, lymph, and other systems. People reach the rhythm of coherence when meditating or through being fully present with the "now." It is a way of focusing the mind and connecting it with your heart.

Brain and body coherence studies have shown that coherence is a healing, restorative state that reduces pain and increases proper body function. Coherence will increase oxygen flow to your head and allow you to be in a state of rest and renew for healing.

The HeartMath Institute developed a small device people can wear to show them when their body and brain are in a state of coherence. This device is designed to help people learn how to achieve this state through feedback from the device.

You can learn more about the device through this link: https://store.heartmath.com/emwave2.

Connect With Others

Connecting with people also helps. We have become a society of disconnection, living alone or texting instead of visiting each other. Helpful hormones are released when we spend time with others.

Generally, your body will go into rest and digest around people who support you. This promotes circulation and all forms of well-being.

Control your thoughts toward the positive as much as possible. Love your life, feel gratitude, feel calm and relaxed, and extend love to your family or friends. Include sex and love with your partner to increase health on many levels.

Daily Relaxation Practices

Avoid long-term sitting. If you work at a computer each day, stopping once an hour to stretch and do slow, deep breathing or walk around a bit is hugely valuable. Limit the hours you spend with blue light electronics. Blue light emitted from cell phones, TVs, computers, and energy-efficient lighting (compact fluorescents and LEDs) can disrupt your circadian rhythm, especially at night, and decrease melatonin production.[15] Melatonin is the "sleep hormone" that also helps the body combat stress and has been linked to the immune system as well.[16] Too many hours with a computer is taxing to the nervous system and can trigger the stress response. Balance in all things promotes better health and feeling energized.

Practicing Qigong works wonders to bring the body into a parasympathetic state, which is just the shift you need to calm the body and supply the brain with more oxygen. One way to quickly relax muscles and relieve pain is to saturate the body with oxygen. This mean lots of air moving in and out, without doing active or strenuous exercise, which will use up the oxygen. Just fill the body with lots of oxygen and many problems will resolve, including muscle tension. Deep belly breathing works as well for this. Take 10 minutes or more to breathe deep into your belly, using your diaphragm to draw air into your lower lungs while your belly rises with each breath. Combine Qigong breathing exercises and hold the relaxation wrist points. These two practices work rapidly, relieving tension and pain in 10 minutes very effectively.

What to do in a traumatic situation: When a migraine comes from a sudden trauma, such as learning of the injury or death of a loved one, feelings can overwhelm the body and cause a massive migraine. Breathe, tune into the body, and do the Stop, Drop, Roll, and Smile protocol, even when smiling is the last thing you want to do. Feel gratitude for anything you can be grateful for in the moment. This will replace some of the large amounts of cortisol running through your systems with serotonin, so you can think more clearly, reduce the pain, and cope with the stressful situation at hand. In this situation, distraction, sleep, or pleasure can help rebalance the body to reduce the pain.

Relaxation Requires Two Steps

The first step is reducing the causes of tension and stress, as described in the previous sections. Second, you will need to increase activities that help you relax. Here are a few valuable activities that help with relaxation:

- Massage
- Qigong
- Thoughtful belly (deep) breathing
- Laughter
- Shaking your whole body, gently or strongly
- Dancing to music
- Yoga or stretching
- Meditation
- Walking in nature
- Quiet, soothing, restful activities
- Help from family and friends, loving support, and understanding

There are many more. Write down the ones that work for you and make time in your life for them, regularly.

Other things you can do on a regular basis include these:

- Get good sleep each night.
- Try NLP (neuro-linguistic programming) to relax around your migraine triggers.
- Get regular exercise.

Diana's Story

When I first started to heal my liver, blood vessels, and neck, and I still had occasional migraines, it was difficult for me to realize my daily life choices were a part of the problem. At the time I was working hard to reach new goals—working into the evening, never taking time to listen to music—and it had become harder for me to meditate. I didn't realize that I was breathing shallowly most of the time.

I couldn't see it then, but I believe now that self-imposed pressure to succeed caused me to live more in fight or flight with less rest-and-digest time for healing. Also, perhaps my liver toxicity, weakened blood vessels, and pinched nerves in my neck caused me to feel as if there was an emergency. Regardless of the cause, learning to consciously relax, to not take success so seriously, and to be present in the moment has allowed me to completely heal.

In Conclusion: Stress

When your migraines are caused by stress, healing can take the form of exploring your personal beliefs, attitudes, and culture around how you view and live your life. This can be difficult and may require the help of others close to you as you try to understand why you react the way you do. You can reach out for professional counseling, life coaching, or the help of a healing practitioner as well, if needed.

Healing from the stress of negative thoughts and emotions can change your outlook on your life—it can help you find forgiveness and see yourself from a broader viewpoint—and you can be happier, on a daily basis, as a result.

Your Future Can Be Free of Migraine and Headache Pain

My healing journey has also been a journey of personal growth, and I suspect it will be for you too. Working to find what helps you relax, what brings a genuine smile to your face, and what brings your body into rest and digest is definitely a learning process, and so worth it—you will benefit from improved health along with freedom from head pain.

I learned about myself and how my attitudes and expectations for my life have affected my health. One of my lessons was that my happiness is not achieved just through my personal success goals—or, more accurately, my personal success goals have changed and now include how I impact others. Taking more time to do the things I love has been part of the journey. Writing this book was one of those things.

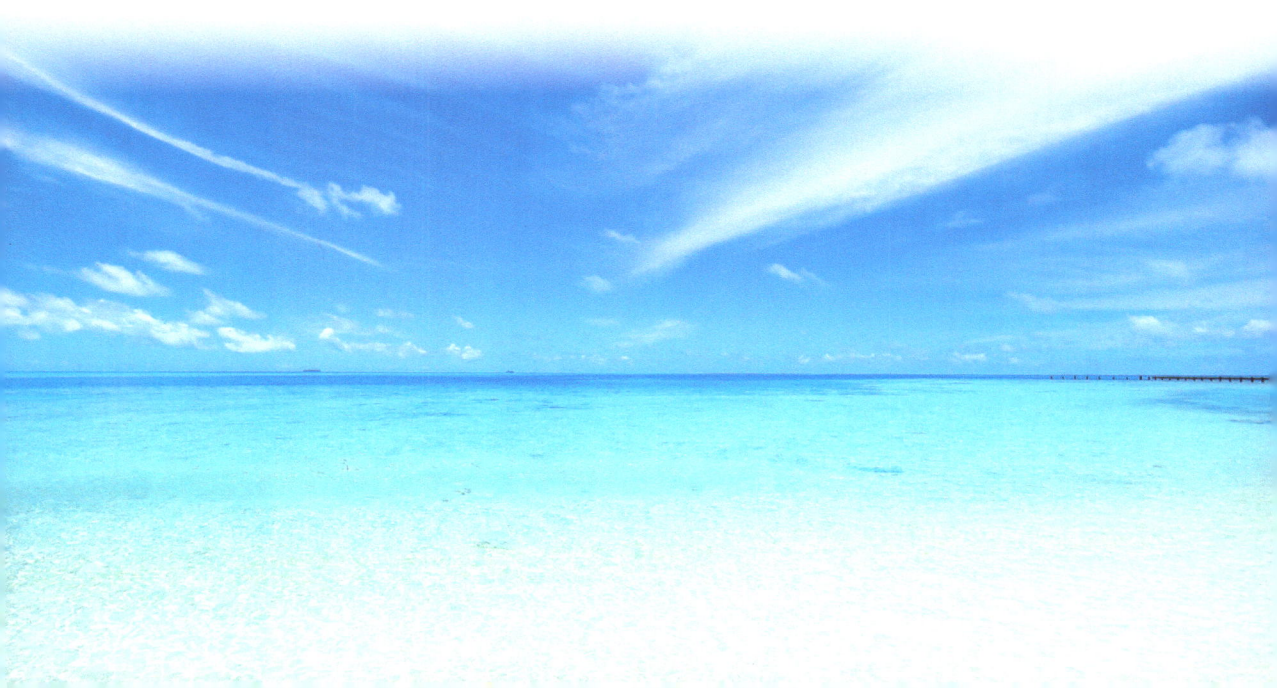

I am still learning and searching for new things that bring me joy—and one of those is helping others learn how to heal their own headache pain so they can live a happier life.

This debilitating pain could be gone forever from your life, if you commit to taking this journey and find the methods and attitudes that work for you and help your body to heal. And once you achieve freedom from head pain, I hope you will join me in sharing what you've learned with others. It will surely make the world a better place.

As of this writing, I am migraine-free and have been completely free for one year, with significant improvements during the two years prior to complete healing. Since I started sharing what I know, I have seen these protocols help many, many others—so I know these steps address widespread issues and not just mine. I am so happy to be free of that pain and I want to share my joy with you to help you find your own path to health

Appendix

The following food lists are provided as guidelines only. Experiment with what works for you.

BLOOD-THICKENING FOODS TO AVOID

Foods High in Vitamin K

Food, amount	Units of Vitamin K/serving
Kale, cooked 1/2 cup	531
Spinach, cooked 1/2 cup	444
Collards, cooked 1/2 cup	418
Swiss chard, raw 1 cup	299
Swiss chard, cooked 1/2 cup	287
Mustard greens, raw 1 cup	279
Turnip greens, cooked 1/2 cup	265
Parsley, raw 1/4 cup	246
Broccoli, cooked 1 cup	220
Brussels sprouts, cooked 1 cup	219
Mustard greens, cooked 1/2 cup	210
Collards, raw 1 cup	184
Spinach, raw 1 cup	145
Turnip greens, raw 1 cup	138
Endive, raw 1 cup	116

Foods High in Saturated Fat

Fatty beef

Lamb

Pork

Poultry with skin

Beef fat (tallow)

Lard and cream

Butter

Cheese

Other dairy products made from whole or 2-percent milk

Cheese substitutes and butter substitutes may be high also

Some baked goods

Fried foods

Palm oil

Palm kernel oil

Coconut (not coconut water)

Coconut oil

Some fermented food

Yogurt (full fat)

Chocolate (as bars or with other saturated fats, especially with added dairy fat)

Other Foods to Avoid During Liver Healing

Pickled foods

Excessive caffeine

Sodium nitrites (in cured meats)

Monosodium glutamate (MSG)

Shellfish, ocean bottom-feeders

All alcohol

FOODS WITH A NEUTRAL EFFECT ON BLOOD

Foods Low in Vitamin K

Food, amount	Units of Vitamin K/serving
Broccoli, raw 1 cup	89
Cabbage, cooked 1/2 cup	82
Green leaf lettuce 1 cup	71
Prunes, stewed 1 cup	65
Romaine lettuce, raw 1 cup	57
Asparagus, 4 spears	48
Avocado, 1 cup	30-48
Tuna, canned in oil 3 ounces	37
Blue- or blackberries, raw 1 cup	29
Peas, cooked 1 cup	41

BLOOD-THINNING FOODS & SUPPLEMENTS TO EAT

Spices

Curry powder
Cayenne pepper
Ginger
Paprika
Thyme
Cinnamon
Dill
Oregano
Turmeric
Licorice
Peppermint

Lake trout
Herring

Fruits

Raisins
Prunes (in moderation, see in Low
Vitamin K list above)
Cherries
Cranberries
Blueberries
Grapes
Strawberries
Tangerines
Oranges
Watermelon
Cantaloupe

Vitamins & Supplements

Vitamin E
Vitamin B6
Vitamin B2
Vitamin D
Omega-3 oils

Fish

Anchovies
Salmon
Albacore tuna
Mackerel

Peaches
Fruits high in moisture

Vegetables

Onions
Celery
Garlic

Liquids

Water
Pure fruit juice
Coconut water
Herbal tea in small quantities,
    because it can be a diuretic

SOURCES

Supplements

Colloidal minerals such as NOW brand, available in health nutrition centers and online, including Amazon: https://smile.amazon.com/NOW-Colloidal-Minerals-Liquid-32-Ounce/dp/B0013OXCU2/ref=sr_1_3?crid=33UL1JWSJ UIKV&keywords=now+colloidal+minerals+liquid%2C32-ounce&qid=1558 018315&s=hpc&sprefix=now+colloidal+%2Chpc%2C236&sr=1-3

Muscle Relaxing Creams and Oils

White Flower Essential Oils – This link is for three bottles, which I always buy because I use this a lot, but you can also buy one bottle at a time on Amazon or your local health food store. https://smile.amazon.com/White-Flower-Balm-Oil-20ml/dp/B01CTFRA74/ref=sr_1_3?crid=2WNG2YL0HJ GH&keywords=white+flower+essential+oil&qid=1558017161&s=hpc&spref ix=white+flower+esse%2Chpc%2C194&sr=1-3

Oil-Free Arnica Liniment with ginger. This has a mild scent and works well also. https://smile.amazon.com/SUPER-SALVE-Arnica-Liniment-FZ/dp/ B014Q32G1W/ref=smi_www_rco2_go_smi_g3905707922?_encoding=UT F8&%2AVersion%2A=1&%2Aentries%2A=0&ie=UTF8

Castor Oil – Topical use for relief of muscle pain.

Some of the links in this book are for products and services I have personally used, and I recommend them. I may be paid a small commission on some products as an affiliate. Please utilize the services of medical professionals and recognize that each product you choose to use is your own decision based on information you gather and your own experience.

Endnotes

1. Https://migraineresearchfoundation.org/about-migraine/migraine-facts/

2. Https://www.mayoclinic.org/medical-professionals/neurology-neurosurgery/news/complexities-of-low-csf-volume-headache/mac-20429665

3. Https://www.ncbi.nlm.nih.gov/pmc/articles/PMC3201065/

4. Https://schott.blogs.nytimes.com/2009/09/23/email-apnea/; https://gizmodo.com/i-stop-breathing-when-i-type-and-you-probably-do-too-1456397692; https://www.businessinsider.com/screen-apnea-2013-9; https://lindastone.net/tag/screen-apnea/

5. Https://www.ncbi.nlm.nih.gov/pmc/articles/PMC5786912/

6. Https://www.ucsfhealth.org/education/heart_disease/; https://www.health.harvard.edu/blog/fda-strengthens-warning-that-nsaids-increase-heart-attack-and-stroke-risk-201507138138

7. Https://www.webmd.com/hypertension-high-blood-pressure/qa/what-are-the-three-main-types-of-blood-vessels; https://www.innerbody.com/image_lymp01/card66.html; Https://my.clevelandclinic.org/health/articles/17059-how-does-blood-flow-through-your-body

8. Https://www.verywellhealth.com/can-opioids-cause-heart-problems-4134144; https://www.uptodate.com/contents/nsaids-adverse-cardiovascular-effects; https://aanmc.org/news/4-reasons-cautious-nsaids/

9. Https://disa.com/map-of-marijuana-legality-by-state

10. Https://www.usatoday.com/story/news/nation-now/2018/06/26/fda-approves-first-cbd-oil-derived-marijuana-treat-epilepsy/733567002/

11. Https://www.inverse.com/article/55030-cbd-could-help-deliver-chemotherapy-drugs; https://www.analyticalcannabis.com/news/break-through-in-cannabinoid-drug-delivery-may-enhance-medical-use-of-cbd-297897; https://www.drugabuse.gov/publications/research-reports/marijuana/how-does-marijuana-produce-its-effects

12. Https://www.ncbi.nlm.nih.gov/pmc/articles/PMC2931553/pdf/bph0160-0523.pdf

13. Cannabinoids and pain: https://www.ncbi.nlm.nih.gov/pmc/articles/PMC3820295/l; Neurological benefits of phytocannabinoids: https://www.ncbi.nlm.nih.gov/pmc/articles/PMC5938896/

14. Https://www.ncbi.nlm.nih.gov/pubmed/20409317

15. Https://www.health.harvard.edu/staying-healthy/blue-light-has-a-dark-side

16. Https://www.ncbi.nlm.nih.gov/pubmed/3327818; Review of melatonin production and receptor sites in immune cells along with most body organs: https://www.ncbi.nlm.nih.gov/pmc/articles/PMC5405617/; Melatonin is created from serotonin: https://www.ncbi.nlm.nih.gov/pmc/articles/PMC4334454/

Resources

Information about the HeartMath Institute's body coherence device can be found here: https://store.heartmath.com/emwave2

BOOKS

William, Anthony. *Medical Medium Liver Rescue: Answers to Eczema, Psoriasis, Diabetes, Strep, Acne, Gout, Bloating, Gallstones, Adrenal Stress, Fatigue, Fatty Liver, Weight Issues, SIBO & Autoimmune Disease* (Hay House Inc., 2018).

Acknowledgments

I would like to thank my mother, Tina Montee, for always being the first person to read and edit my books and fix the typos so I can feel confident enough to let others read them. She is a far better writer than I and everything about her life inspires me to live more fully and be more like her. I would like to thank my aunt Carla Siebel for always being the second person to read my books and find many ways I could improve them. Together they have lovingly and politely read many early drafts of my several works.

I am grateful for my dear sister, Jina Nelson, for her confidence in me, as well as her genuine support and encouragement. My three daughters, Rebecca Kent, Christina Bartschi, and Shari DeVaard, always offer me their love and confidence. Their bright, beautiful spirits give me all of the motivation I need. Thank you, my sweet daughters. I do nothing in this world without keeping you in mind!

With very few words, my father, Ken Montee, believes in me and wants nothing more than for me to receive what I desire. Thank you, Dad.

Thank you to my dear friends. Julie Lynn, for her confidence and support and for sharing how she healed herself from migraines with willpower and belief. She is a strong, incredible woman. Thanks to Narda Pitkethly for believing in me, giving me advice and support. Narda's personal accomplishments show me that one person can make a tremendous difference in the world. I have many other amazing friends who have inspired me along the way:

Jody Stanislaw, Julie Johnson, Kristen Schneck, Lynnette Jones, Ashiauna Louderbough, and Ann Peach.

I wish to thank several doctors for their contribution to my long-term health. My dear Dr. Michael Moriarty, who became my friend after putting me back together as my chiropractor for 35 years, following four separate car accidents. He started me on the path to understanding healing the body and good health practices. Dr. Steve Politis, who did minute adjustments in my neck to free up more blood traveling to my brain. I am forever grateful for his expertise and excellent training. He also reminded me to belly breathe when I had forgotten. Dr. Bart Goldman, who read my early draft of the full book and gave me his expert opinion and blessing. Bart was a great resource from the medical per-spective. My heartfelt thanks to Dr. Erik Jones for alerting me to the dangers of opiate painkillers. He helped me take one of my most significant steps on my healing journey and opened my eyes to the harm these medications cause.

Then I come to my blessed publishing team. I greatly appreciate Maryanna Young for taking an interest in my project and publishing the first products, such as this one. Maryanna is a visionary and expert in her industry. Of course, I could not have created a concise, logical structure without my fabulous editor, Jennifer Regner. She is brilliant at what she does.

I appreciate all the wonderful people in my life who have crossed my path or supported me. There are too many to name. Thankfully we don't travel this world alone. This material would not be available without the energy of many other beings, including all of those with migraines who allowed me to share this information to help them on their journey. I appreciate *all* the individuals who helped this work become available.

About the Author

Diana Anderson lived with migraine headaches for her entire adult life, until the prescribed medications no longer relieved her pain. She also realized her headaches had been increasing in severity and frequency and she had more triggers than ever before—including being at higher altitudes and wearing a hat. She researched alternatives and sought out practitioners to help her regain her health. Over the course of almost three years, her learning journey brought her to a new understanding that migraine headaches were an indicator that something in the body needed healing. After healing herself, her intimate knowledge of migraine pain motivated her to write her knowledge down so she could share it and help others.

Diana is not content to lie still and watch the world happen around her. She enjoys experiencing life to the fullest and creating powerful memories. When migraines took the joy of life from her, she was absolutely determined to get her spark back.

Now that she has her spark back, she enjoys traveling the world, hiking, biking, floating the rivers, and spending time in the solitude of nature. When she is not in her flower garden, she is with friends or family, writing at her computer, or exploring this glorious planet. When given the opportunity, she also teaches at retreats, workshops, and courses about the tools she has found useful to enjoy a healthy, fulfilled life.

Her five grandkids call her Nana and they ride on her back, chase her around at the zoo, and help her tend to the garden. She is thankful for so many of life's unlimited wonders and the inspiring people around her. However, her greatest joys come from her family, especially her three brilliant daughters, her delightful, energetic grandkids, and her sons-in-law. She lives in Idaho, surrounded by the outdoors she loves to explore.

Diana is a prolific author. If you want to connect with her other products, see the list below. She has written two novels and three books for women on improving intimate pleasure with a partner. She has a course for men and a course for women on how to improve the connection in the bedroom as well as the pleasure and fun.

If you would like to contact Diana about a speaking or teaching engagement on the topic of migraines, health, or pleasure, reach out to her on her website, RealMigraineSolutions.com.

CONNECT WITH ME

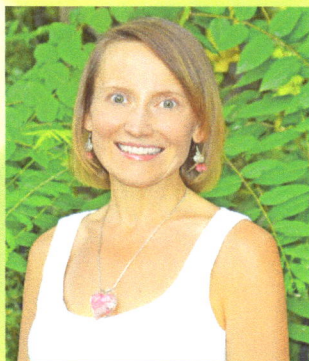

If this book helped you, I would love to hear from you. Connect with me on my Facebook group, on my Facebook page, on LinkedIn, or contact me through my website at RealMigraineSolutions.com.

Please share this information with anyone you know who suffers from headaches or migraines. Let others know how it helped you by posting a review on Amazon or Goodreads or by spreading the word on social media.

My hope is to reach as many people as possible with these simple steps toward making their lives better and less painful.

Be well. I hope your life is full of joy.

Diana Anderson

RealMigraineSolutions.com

Facebook group: Facebook.com/group/realmigrainesolutions/

Facebook: Facebook.com/dianamonteeanderson

LinkedIn: Diana Anderson, https://www.linkedin.com/in/Diana-Anderson-96b07219/

www.ingramcontent.com/pod-product-compliance
Lightning Source LLC
Chambersburg PA
CBHW060810270326

41928CB00003B/50